PLAY TO WIN THE FOOD FIGHT

Jim,

I hope this book brings guidance & encouragement

PLAY TO WIN THE FOOD FIGHT

By
Reshaunda Thornton, MS, RD, LD, CSSD

St. Louis, Missouri • 2019

Copyright © 2019 by Reshaunda Thornton.

All rights reserved. No part of this publication may be reproduced, stored in a retrieval system, or transmitted in any form or by any means, electronic, mechanical, photocopying, recording, or otherwise, without prior permission of the author.

Printed in the United States of America

The author has, as far as possible, taken every precaution to ensure that the information given in this text is accurate and up to date. The author will not be responsible for any errors or omissions or liable for actions taken as a result of information or opinions expressed in this book. Names have been changed for privacy purposes. No liability is assumed for damages that may result from the use of information contained within.

ISBN: 978-0-578-22429-9

*To my son, John Tristan Edwards, Jr.
Always remember to find your own path to what makes you great.
Then, lead and be a gift to others.*

FORWARD

After being in the industry for almost 15 years, I have become acquainted with many fellow dietitians, but none are quite like Reshaunda Thornton. Hearing Reshaunda share her expertise on nutrition and the daily pitfalls that come with attempting to lead a healthy lifestyle is refreshing, as many unqualified self-proclaimed gurus are misinforming the public and creating greater harm than good.

There is so much information on the Internet about health and nutrition that it can be utterly confusing for the person starting their health and fitness journey. While there are some great resources on health and nutrition that can easily be searched, there are also numerous non-science-based materials that can be misleading and be detrimental to a person's health.

For these reasons, I am ecstatic that Reshaunda has written *Play to Win the Food Fight* about how to win the war against the temptations and struggles that most people face when making food choices.

As the "anti-diet" dietitian, Reshaunda reveals in this book some of the key principles that many people are missing in their quest for a healthy lifestyle, and if we are honest, the best body they can have.

This book is not based on what the author thinks but rather is grounded in the many years of research and client interactions that have led her to conclude that a healthy eating plan doesn't start with just the food that you eat. Instead, it's the mindset you have before starting.

What is unique about this book is that Reshaunda doesn't just give you a list of foods you should or should not eat. Instead, she challenges you to do the deep work and get in tune with your relationship with food. She challenges you to confront your views about food and gives you action steps at the end of each chapter to help you put into practice what you have learned.

Play to Win the Food Fight is not just a resource for the person who seeks to improve their health. This book will also be a valuable go-to resource for dietitians and nutrition professionals as we help our clients reach the goals they deserve.

Now that you are ready to do the work, take control of your health, and be the best version of yourself for those who depend on you, dive into this book. Reshaunda maps out a process that will lead you directly to your health and fitness goals.

Percy Bass RD, CPT
Owner of Head2Toe Fitness Studio
www.h2tfitness.com
www.h2tzone.com

FORWARD

In a time when people are more confused than ever about nutrition, Reshaunda Thornton offers a comprehensive, straightforward solution to help folks gain clarity and win the food fight — for good.

So many nutrition books focus on which foods are "good" or "bad," "on plan" or "off," "allowed" or "forbidden." This rigid, black-and-white thinking is why so many people spend their life on the diet roller coaster.

You won't find any of that in this book.

Reshaunda understands that nourishing our bodies and having a healthy relationship with food is about much more than simply following a diet.

In *Play to Win the Food Fight*, Reshaunda discusses all the critical topics affecting our food choices and behaviors, including our environment, our emotional connection to food, finding our *Why*, our patterns and rituals, how we self-sabotage, and more.

A few years ago, when I first learned of Reshaunda's work through our mutual friend, Kourtney Thomas, I knew she was special. Not only does she have an impressive formal education, but she also has personal experience as an athlete. With her well-rounded approach to nutrition, she has helped countless people change their mindset about healthful eating.

That's why I invited her to be an Academy Curriculum Developer for our Girls Gone Strong Level 1 Coaching Certification — to help educate health and fitness professionals about women-specific health and fitness topics. Now, I'm thrilled her information will reach the masses with this book.

I'm heartened and delighted to see a nutrition book that not only covers the psychological aspects of why we eat the way we do but also provides actionable tools, skills, and information to help readers create the lasting change they crave.

Molly Galbraith
Woman-in-Charge, Girls Gone Strong
Creator, Coaching & Training Women Academy
www.academy.girlsgonestrong.com

FORWARD

It's time for the confusion to end as to why so many people go on a food and emotional roller coaster when it comes to trying to take control of their health. In *Play to Win the Food Fight*, Reshaunda truly captures why many people find the road difficult and gives guidance about how to finally claim the captain's seat. One of the first steps is discovering how our upbringing and environment influence the paths we take in life. Then, Reshaunda gives us tools to arm ourselves, so food and negativity lose their power.

As a wellness specialist for 20 years, I have listened to thousands of clients talk about their fight with weight, their struggles with staying on track, and how they beat themselves up over what they call "bad" eating. This book addresses the power you give the words "good" and "bad" to describe food, suggesting replacements like "unhealthy" and "healthy." By making simple word changes, one can connect honestly to what will give their bodies lifelong benefits.

Play To Win the Food Fight also drives home the importance of knowing the life you have been leading and how to begin anew. Knowledge comes from educating yourself on what's really in food, taking the time to read labels, and understanding what holds you back from living your best life. The marketing ploys that elevate healthy-appearing food has also led to distrust. Reshaunda puts you in control once and for all, ensuring you understand clean and whole food options and how not to give in to the countless fast and convenient food options.

Reshaunda and I have worked together with clients over the years. The comment I hear most is how she simplifies what has led to the pounds, the self-sabotage, and the challenge of finding happiness within. She has a real connection with her clients and uncovers those *ah-ha* moments they need for lifelong success.

This book will be a welcome addition to those building a healthier foundation, healing past wounds, and reversing the damage that prevents them from living the life they have always wanted.

Monica Adams, PT
FOX 2 News in the Morning Anchor
Wellness and Transformation Specialist

PREFACE

Have you looked at old pictures and thought about how much smaller you were or how different life was? Perhaps you look back and you've been in the same place for the past 10 years? Can you picture a time when your health was at its optimum and the freedom that came with it? Maybe you've spent hundreds of dollars on not one but several programs that haven't delivered on their promise of quick-fix results.

If this sounds like you, you're not alone. As a registered dietitian in private practice, I've worked with hundreds of clients who struggle with losing weight and making healthier nutritional choices as they navigate through life's constant changes.

This book is a culmination of the lessons, revelations that have surprised me, and strategies I've shared with my clients.

If you're looking for a book that provides food portions for weight loss, the healthiest recipes, or the best cookie-cutter diet approach, you won't find that kind of advice within these pages.

Instead, this book begins by addressing the underlying influences about why you may lack control with specific foods and why you've failed in the past. This battle is one that many people face. While the fight is bigger than food, it's not bigger than you! To help you win the battle, I delve into the emotional attachments around food and provide strategies for breaking patterns.

I focus on getting down to what may be holding you back, keeping you stuck, making you sick, contributing to long-term issues, affecting your self-esteem, and causing you to lose confidence during your journey. If you've had trouble dieting, keeping weight off, or are plagued with health conditions that are affected or reflected by poor habits or relationships with food, you've come to the right place.

Sound like a tall task? Don't feel overwhelmed.

I've intentionally divided this book into seven parts with 32 easy-to-digest chapters. You will find mantras at the start of each chapter to serve as inspiration. Additionally, I've scattered throughout the book several client success stories. I hope that their words will resonate with your experiences, and you will find yourself saying, *"that sounds like me"* or *"I never thought about it like that."*

Because I'm a dietitian, you can expect to find nuggets of nutrition wisdom embedded in this book. But I also wanted to leave you with more than my words on the page. To make this book most useful, at the end of chapters I've included game plans called *How to Win*. In these, I give take-away advice about strategies you can do right now to shift your mindset and overcome obstacles as you transition to healthier choices.

When you are finished, you will know how to break down and build a healthier relationship with food. You will be more confident, self-aware, and empowered, so you won't think twice about saying no to the persons, places, or things that have been holding you back from making lasting change.

I'm so glad you're here. Be ready to make changes, shift your mindset, and transform into the person you were meant to be.

Reshaunda Thornton, MS, RD, LD, CSSD

ACKNOWLEDGMENTS

Before anything, I would like to thank God. You have given me the power to believe in my passion and pursue my dreams. Without faith, this would not have been possible.

Writing a book was only a "good idea" that has turned into a fulfilling project that can impact more lives. Now, I understand the work and energy it takes to put years and passion on paper. Thank you Envision By Design for taking the lead in editing, designing the book, and taking it to print. Your work shows for itself.

CONTENTS

Forewords   *Percy Bass RD, CPT*   vii
            Molly Galbraith   ix
            Monica Adams, PT   xi

PART I   Getting Ready
1 Uncovering Environmental Influences   3
2 Understanding the Nutrition Lingo   7
3 Are You Making Excuses?   13
4 No More "Diet" Mentality   15
5 Are You in Opposition or Partnership?   19

PART II   Strategies for Winning
6 Find Your *Why*   27
7 Are You Fighting a Repeat Weight-Loss Battle?   31
8 Food Wears Many Hats, But Which Hat It Wears Is Up to You   37
9 You Are the Driver in Charge   41
10 Building Better Confidence   45
11 The Point of No Return   49

PART III   Preparing for Challenges
12 Patterns, Patterns, Patterns!   55
13 Associations and Attachments   59
14 Things Pop Up! What Are You Going to Do?   65

PART IV   Know Your Allies and Opponents
15 You Need Water   73
16 Knock Out Empty Calorie Options   75

17 The Unholy Trinity of Preservatives:
    Fat, Sugar, Sodium   79
18 Eat Like Your Metabolism   83
19 Facing Temptations: Second (and Third) Helpings   87
20 Final Nuts and Bolts   91

PART V   Six Game Plans That Really Work
21 #1 Challenges Are Inevitable – You'll Prevail   97
22 #2 Practice Means Progress   99
23 #3 Reposition Yourself   101
24 #4 See Food Not as a Tool But as Nutrition   103
25 #5 Know the Difference: Food vs. Nutrition   105
26 #6 Give Yourself Validation   107

PART VI   What It Takes to Win
27 Motivation Is A Good Starter, But …   111
28 Pursue Consistency   115

PART VII   Inspiration for Fighting Your Best Fight
29 My Hope for You Is Liberation   121
30 You've Got One Shot!   125
31 Once You've Learned to Fish – Keep Fishing   127
32 I Believe in You   133

PLAY TO WIN THE FOOD FIGHT

PART I
Getting Ready

Uncovering Environmental Influences

Understanding the Nutrition Lingo

Saying Goodbye to Excuses

Eliminating the Diet Mentality

Knowing the Connection Between Emotions and Food

"We can't be afraid of change. You may feel very secure in the pond that you are in, but if you never venture out of it, you will never know that there is such a thing as an ocean, a sea. Holding onto something that is good for you now, may be the very reason why you don't have something better."

C. JoyBell C.

CHAPTER 1

UNCOVERING ENVIRONMENTAL INFLUENCES

"Be aware of your environment, and its impact on your choices."

Your environment can be determined by many factors, including geography, economics, and culture. Culture is a "way of life" for groups of people, meaning the way they do things. Different groups may have different cultures. Cultural habits are often passed on through generations. Since we inherit them, we may not recognize how we are influenced by our surroundings or environment when we make our choices.

For example, many people in New York City walk or take public transportation to get to their destination. Many city dwellers don't have vehicles of their own as a result. When it's time for groceries, many go the closest bodega (little corner store) and purchase their meals on the spot. Or they buy groceries daily in small quantities so they are easier to carry. Makes sense, right? However, in the suburb of Houston, where I grew up, almost everyone has cars, and large grocery stores are the norm. On any given day, parking lots are full of mini-vans filled with families loading their weeks-worth of groceries. These environments are incredibly different, yet the differences may not seem relevant or apparent. But recognizing what's happening around you can make all the difference when working to make significant changes in food choices and lifestyle.

THE RELATIONSHIP BETWEEN ENVIRONMENT AND CHOICES

Your environment impacts your choices and decisions. Think about it. If you were raised in a family that cooks rich and high-calorie foods, you are accustomed to this specific taste and cooking technique. If your family typically eats fast food or frozen meals for dinner, transitioning into preparing home-cooked meals may be difficult. If you grew up in an area where few grocery stores sold fresh produce, you might not be accustomed to eating it. Furthermore, you might find it challenging to incorporate whole foods (perishables like produce and meats), into your everyday eating.

Many times variables like these that play a role in our upbringing affect us as adults and influence the choices we make.

 HOW TO WIN! Overcome Environmental Influences

Has your environment unknowingly played a role in your decision-making? What we eat is often a result of what we are presented with. Recognizing these factors gives you the power to make new choices.

The following statements will raise your awareness and help you beat outside influences:
- Recognize that you have choices when it comes to what you eat.
- Know that you may have been influenced to eat a certain food.
- Quick does not mean quality.
- When grocery shopping, try to stay in the "outer ring" where stores locate fruits, vegetables, lean meats, fish, eggs, and nuts.
- Rethink, "say no to temptation" (see Chapter 19).
- Don't push the better choice to another day. Make your best choice today.

- Distance yourself when you feel cravings. You usually know when they will strike and can prepare.
- Think about unhealthy food differently. What effect will it have on your body?
- Visualize the negative consequences, and then visualize the positive consequences of your choices.
- Surround yourself with healthy food options so you can make better choices.
- Remember, positive energy comes from positive choices, and negative energy comes from negative choices. Whenever possible, choose positive energy.

CHAPTER 2

UNDERSTANDING THE NUTRITION LINGO

"Just when you think you are eating healthy, a new tabloid headline makes you second guess yourself."

If you are like most people, you have been bombarded throughout your life with information about what is healthy only to find out it is the worst thing for you. For example, when I was growing up, we were encouraged to drink milk, and now researchers and doctors say milk is unhealthy for adults. We also grew up with the food pyramid emphasizing high grain intake. Today, the industry is saying *"grains/breads are our worst enemy."*

Conflicting information makes us suspicious about who to trust and what to do. Especially if you don't have a "why" behind what's "good" or "bad." When you are shopping and see a label that says "pure" or "high in protein," do you really know what that means? It's all confusing. You might be left feeling unsure about your choices. And when you feel uncertain about something, it's easy to give up, saying you'll try again, another time.

I'm not telling you to take college courses on nutrition and dietetics. Your interest level may not reach that far, and it's okay. It is more important to pick up some basics, learn as you go, and ask questions when in doubt. As you build your knowledge-base and confidence, you create a foundation for continued learning.

THE FOOD INDUSTRY SKEWS OUR PERSPECTIVE

The food industry uses marketing to drive sales and to increase revenue, at the cost of consumers' best interest. Profit takes priority over nutritional benefits, and we all suffer as a result. That influence has taken us so far from "real" food that our taste buds are desensitized to whole foods. Everything is made cheap and fast, packaged for convenience, and processed. We are left with cheese products instead of real cheese and meat products rather than real meat.

The food industry created fast food as an answer to our fast-paced lifestyles. Driving down a typical, populated road, you are bound to find restaurants and gas stations promising convenient or packaged food, quickly. The message is, *"You need food fast. We're your answer!"* It's easy to be persuaded and find justification. Before you know it, you, just like many of us, become subject to what they offer. You sacrifice quickness for nutrients.

WHAT DO THE WORDS MEAN?

Understanding food terms as well as what's in the food you eat can help you make healthier choices. This knowledge also makes it easier to compare different options.

Clean Food. Food in its most natural state without any extra ingredients or processing. For example, peanut butter should contain only peanuts. Oatmeal should contain only oats. Food in this category includes unrefined grains, fresh or frozen fruits and vegetables, and unprocessed meat. Furthermore, clean food minimizes canning, jarring, bottling, and boxing. If you see a box of food on a shelf, it's probably not clean food.

Complex Carbohydrates (also known as "good" carbs). Your body uses carbohydrates for energy. Complex carbs are digested more slowly than simple carbs and leave you feeling satisfied for a more extended period. Complex carbs are found in whole grains, (breads, pasta, crackers), beans, fruit, oatmeal, sweet potatoes, and corn.

Complex carbs can help lower glycemic levels, provide fiber, and slow digestion. They help you feel content and energized.

Fiber (also known as "roughage"). Fiber comes from plant food that we don't digest because we don't have the necessary enzymes. Fiber provides our bodies with tons of nutrients. The best sources of fiber are found in fruits, vegetables, whole grains, and legumes.

Fruits. Fresh or frozen fruits contain essential nutrients like potassium and fiber as well as antioxidants. Some of the healthiest fruits to eat include grapefruit, blackberries, raspberries, blueberries, apples, pomegranates, mangos, strawberries, lemons, melons, oranges, bananas, grapes, and cherries. Whenever possible, avoid fruit with added sugar.

Healthy Fats (also known as "good" fats). Not all fat is bad for you, and fat is necessary to absorb vitamins and to protect your brain and heart. Good fats are plant- and fish-based. Healthy fats include unsaturated fats, monounsaturated fats, polyunsaturated fats, and omega-3 fatty acids. Foods that contain healthy fat include seeds, olives, avocados, nuts, nut butters, plant-based oils (olive, flaxseed, and coconut), and fatty fish.

"Bad" fats include trans fat and saturated fats which can contribute to an increased risk for certain diseases. Foods containing these types of fats are typically animal-based. They can be found in packaged pastries, stick margarine or shortening, fried foods, red meat (beef, lamb, and pork), butter, and ice cream (see Chapter 17).

Non-perishable Snacks. These healthier food choices can be prepared in advance and used for tasty treats in between meals. The best snacks are nuts, pretzels, (air-popped) popcorn, granola bars, individual portion packs of whole-grain crackers, dry roasted snacks, or nut- and fruit-based trail mix.

Organic Food. Food produced without man-made fertilizers and pesticides or genetically modified organisms (GMOs). There are different organic standards throughout the world.

Protein (lean). Protein provides the essential building blocks of what your body needs to thrive and helps to increase your immune system. The best options for lean protein can be found in fish, chicken breast, turkey breast, 93% or higher ground meat (beef or poultry), beef and pork tenderloin, Canadian bacon, and eggs. Non-animal proteins like soybeans and tofu are also sources of lean protein.

Simple Carbohydrates (also known as "bad" carbs). Simple carbs are refined sugars added to sweeten and increase the shelf life of foods (see Chapter 17). You can find them in processed bread products, white rice, breakfast cereal, pastries, cakes, fruit juices, and soda.

Because simple carbs lack nutrients, they can increase glycemic levels and can lead to chronic health conditions. Try to avoid them and find other options for satisfying sweet cravings. Your body quickly digests simple carbs and converts them into fat after your daily caloric intake has been met.

Vegetables. The nutrients you get from vegetables are essential for good health and can help reduce the risk of chronic conditions. Vegetables are good sources of vitamins, minerals, and fiber. The healthiest veggies include fresh or frozen spinach; dark, green leafy vegetables; broccoli; brussels sprouts; kale; cauliflower; squash; and asparagus. Whenever possible, avoid overcooking vegetables, so they retain their nutritional value and steer clear of canned veggies and those prepared with sauces.

Whole Food. Food mainly from plants that has not been (or minimally) processed. Food in this category include fruits, vegetables, legumes, whole grains, seeds, and nuts.

HOW TO WIN! Tips for Healthy Eating

Making lifestyle changes can be hard. If you are facing challenges for healthier food choices, consider the following tips:
- Choose to eat a fiber-filled diet with whole grains, fruits, and vegetables.
- Select fish, poultry, nuts, and beans for protein.
- Limit foods high in saturated fat and avoid food with trans fat.
- Drink water to quench your thirst and take advantage of additional benefits like improved memory, better immunity, fewer headaches, and regularity (see Chapter 15).
- Grill, bake, or broil food to decrease high-fat calories instead of frying.
- Focus on eating vegetables and protein first during a meal before eating carbohydrates.
- Limit salt intake and select fresh foods over processed foods.
- Mix up foods to try new and different taste sensations.
- Beware of marketing labels like "natural," "light," and "pure." These terms are not federally regulated and might be misleading. When in doubt, read the ingredient list on the food label.

CHAPTER 3

ARE YOU MAKING EXCUSES?

"Pause to step back and recognize what it is that has been holding you back, slowing you down, or stopping you. Whatever it is, acknowledge it, and stop making excuses."

We use excuses to rationalize our actions about circumstances, decisions, and events. Furthermore, **excuses prevent us from acting and hold us back from opportunities in life.**

Have you been making excuses for moving forward to accomplish your health goals? Maybe these statements have flitted through your brain or have come out of your mouth:
- *"My work schedule is too busy."*
- *"I have too many responsibilities as a parent."*
- *"I need to wait until after this holiday season."*

Take a few moments to stop and assess your choices and the reasons behind them. Then, think about refocusing.

Everyone is faced with challenges that can cause them to lose focus. Events will happen that keep us locked into excuses and procrastination. It's easier to push back, ignore, or deny the changes in your energy level or the extra pounds on the scale. However, if you keep putting off what you could do today, you will have more problems to address in the future. The truth is, there will never be a perfect time to focus on how your health is affected by your food choices.

HOW TO WIN! Committing to Fewer Excuses

If you find yourself drowning in excuses, try these strategies to proactively stop making excuses to get what you want out of life:
- Focus on your *Why* (see Chapter 6).
- Understand that excuses are crutches. They may be dependable. But know that you don't need crutches, and you don't need excuses.
- Recognize negative thoughts will always tell you it's too hard. Drown out the negative voices with your positive actions.
- Say your excuses out loud, write them down, and look at them. How do they look now? If they sound silly or invalid, change them with new choices.
- Decide how long you want to live in a world of excuses. Excuses will never help you advance to where you want to be.
- Think about when you hear your child, spouse, or anyone in your life make excuses. What are the thoughts that run through your head? Do you think, *"They are full of excuses"*? Remember that the next time you catch yourself making excuses!
- Ask yourself, *"what excuses are holding me back?"* Identifying your reasons will help you plan for moving forward.
- Plan for hurdles and challenges, decrease excuses, and focus on solutions and opportunities.
- Focus on your strengths instead of how incapable you might feel. Excuses have the power to make us think that we can't accomplish our goals or make changes.

CHAPTER 4

NO MORE "DIET" MENTALITY

"When you eliminate 'diet,' food doesn't change, but your perspective does. What once was desirable is now unappealing."

WHAT'S WRONG WITH DIETING?
Every day I see people jump on the diet bandwagon because it gives them hope. So, why am I so against diets? I'm against the diet mentality because people feel forced to conform, they are restricted, and many are pressured by unrealistic expectations.

Rather than jumping into diets that promise quick fixes, my wish is for people to stop subscribing to a system of set diet rules they can't wait to break. If you've ever been on a diet, does this sound like you?
- You hate following the rules set by the program.
- You can't wait until you finish.
- You feel disappointed if you don't see quick results.
- You feel hopeless because change is hard.

The diet mentality is one of the battles to win in your struggle with food, and the solution is a change in thinking. Instead of thinking about dieting, I encourage you to begin building a healthy relationship with food.

When you commit to looking at yourself in a relationship with food, you will find that you are also building a healthier relationship with yourself with a focus on health and wellness.

And it works!

WHAT'S BETTER ABOUT A FOOD RELATIONSHIP?

Everything you eat contributes to the deterioration or enhancement of your body. Every choice you make reflects how you feel about yourself. When you decide to eat for your health, you are taking care of yourself – and you feel better. You feel better about the choices you are making and about what you are eating. In the process, you are building awareness and a relationship with yourself and with what you consume.

You are creating a relationship with what you eat to forge a path to a long-lasting and liberating life.

When you create a healthy relationship with food, you are more connected to what you eat as well as who you are. Like any relationship, you seek benefits and security continuously. This collaboration eases stress, helps avoid mental and physical illness, provides energy, and ensures the ability to live a healthy life. All of this starts with you giving your time and attention.

Consider the characteristics of a long-term, positive relationship:
- Creativity
- Disappointments followed by forgiveness
- Caring when you least want to
- Building rapport by learning
- Honesty
- Letting go of perfection

Contrast this with a picture of an unhealthy relationship:
- Feeling a lack of control
- Not caring about your choices
- Ignoring what's most important – your health

All relationships require a sense of presence and awareness. The same is true when you establish a healthy relationship with food. That's why it's important to connect with your food, be true to it, and see yourself in your choices.

What does it take to build a food relationship? You must learn the emotional ties you have to food, understand what your choices reflect, and take time to learn new habits.

> ### 🏆 HOW TO WIN!
> ### Building a Healthy Relationship with Food

One of the first steps to winning the battle over the diet mentality is seeing nutrition as your lifeline and long-term partner that you cannot opt out of!

As you begin building your new food relationships, the following are some of the first steps for looking at food differently:

- Understand your food is your lifeline for survival. Your survival is dependent upon having air to breathe, water to drink, and food to eat. We prefer to breathe fresh, clean air free from pollution. We want to drink filtered, chemical-free water instead of contaminated liquid. Begin holding your food choices to similar standards by fueling your body with the best nutrients. Think about how many times you have chosen a greasy hamburger over a fresh, nutrient-filled apple.

- Realize your food is your lifelong partner. Food is with you longer than any other person or object in your life. And it will help determine your quality of life. You are the one in control of the partnership.

- Recognize that you don't get to opt out of eating. You can decide to go to the gym or stay home, change the radio station if you don't like the song, and change jobs if you are not happy. But when it comes to the food your body needs to survive, you can't opt out.

CHAPTER 5

ARE YOU IN OPPOSITION OR PARTNERSHIP?

"Unknowingly, most of us have an adversarial relationship to food which overpowers our connection with self. It's time to change that.."

IS FOOD RUNNING YOUR LIFE?
How many times have you felt that food has the upper hand and drives your choices? When you smell the chocolate cake, are you under a trance to put a large piece on your plate, thinking that you will be happy when the last forkful is in your mouth? And then you realize that rarely is true happiness at the end of the fork. Instead, you are left feeling regret and failure.

Most of us experience an emotional attachment to food. Food is by your side when you are tired, frustrated, happy, anxious, and even bored. Eating is a constant throughout our lives. You may find almost every emotion you have is connected to food. Instead of ignoring the connections, recognizing them is essential to plan how you will react strategically.

Think about team sports and reruns. When you know the play and have seen the outcome, you are better equipped to win the game. The same is true when playing the game with food, a familiar opponent. If you know the playing field, your emotional connections and reactions, and your strengths and weaknesses, you will have the advantage of winning the battle. You will know what to expect and can position yourself in the offensive position.

Then, you will win the game and successfully build a new relationship with your opponent.

If you're still unsure whether you or food has the upper hand in the game, you wouldn't be the first, and you won't be the last.

That's why it's essential to connect with our inner selves to retain our power. When you have an unhealthy relationship with food, food has control over every choice. Then, you begin believing that you don't have a choice and aren't strong enough to win or change.

THE DOWNFALL OF DEFINING FOOD AS "GOOD" OR "BAD"

Today, a large part of society has identified food as either *good* or *bad*. And we unconsciously put certain foods into one of these two categories. We use "good" or "bad" to deter us from certain foods. Furthermore, the "good" and "bad" word choice can translate into how we define ourselves. How many times have you said, *"I was bad today,"* when referring to the bag of chips you had at lunch? Maybe you've said, *"I was good all day,"* when you resisted the temptation to have second helpings.

When you make these comments, you are defining yourself by your actions and food choices. You've given the food the power position.

Rather than seeing food as good or bad, I think of food as healthy or unhealthy. By making this simple wording change, you articulate how food choices can affect your health.

Why are we defining ourselves by our food choices? The struggle doesn't begin with food; it starts with our emotions.

OUR EMOTIONAL CONNECTION TO FOOD BEGINS IN OUR BRAIN

The brain is a remarkable organ. It can interpret, ration, and distinguish. The interconnected constructions within the limbic system are responsible for our emotions and behaviors. This region is where the conditioned connection between your emotions and food choices originates.

Therefore, every food item you encounter is most likely connected to an emotion stemming from deeply embedded memories. Because of the emotional connections, food becomes your comforter, self-inflictor, the reward, or the "answer" to weight loss and feeling better about yourself.

There is a strong emotional connection to the choices we make with our foods and how we unconsciously feel about ourselves. If we say a particular food is "bad" when we eat it, we are essentially saying we are bad. We become directly connected to what we choose to eat. When we eat bad, we feel bad; we feel guilty; we feel like a failure.

Here's the secret. Break the ties of emotional connections and prevent your food choices from defining who you are right now. Instead, let your food choices define who you *want* to be and what you want for your health and body. Your choices will dictate long-term health benefits.

If you look in the mirror and see a reflection of someone unhappy in their skin, understand that what you see is a by-product of your past choices. The answer to changing your reflection is changing your mindset and addressing the emotional connection you have with food. It's not about putting all your energy into changing only your physical manifestation that you see in your reflection.

Most of us are in the habit of fighting what we see; however, that's not where the real fight starts. Shifting your perspective is about internal change which positions you to live a life defined by positive thoughts of yourself versus food choices.

KAREN'S STORY

When I met Karen, she described the number of diets she'd tried, her weight fluctuations, and her anxiety about trying to change what she saw in the mirror. She talked about how she has never had a feeling of peace, and her weight has been the culprit. In the past, she found herself continually fighting her weight and feeling like a failure every time she gained it back.

Karen was exhausted.

She said it felt like running a marathon on Monday and getting back up to run another marathon on Tuesday. This constant, nonstop battle prevented her from feeling the peace she needed for her life.

We took time to address patterns and emotional connections that led back to unhappy childhood occurrences. We also dealt with her negative self-talk that kept saying she was bound to fail again.

She realized that change started with first recognizing the root cause of her emotions. Then, we began the work of separating how she feels from the natural response of going to food.

I want to say Karen's solution was a quick and easy fix. However, after many years of using food as her scapegoat, we both knew that change would take time and patience. There would also be days of reminding herself that food doesn't have to live in the same space with emotion.

Soon, she began to take the lead in her life. Furthermore, she decided to start dictating how she *wants* to see herself.

As a result of hard work, Karen's food struggle became easier. She gained more confidence as she found control over her actions, and eventually, the peace she was seeking became a reality. Karen found that the more she desired peace, the less she had to fight herself.

Karen still has struggles, as we all do, but now she is better equipped to take the right steps to lead her in the direction she wants to go.

🏆 HOW TO WIN! Moving Into the Offensive Position

Consider the following steps for changing your mindset and breaking the emotional attachment to food.
- Recognize where you are physically and emotionally and if you are where you want to be. If the answer is no, continue reading!
- Take a deep breath and realize what makes you unsettled.
- Create a list of three emotion and food trigger connections. For example, I always craved late-night sweets. I was nervous and ate salty snacks. I felt disappointment and had ice cream. It's Friday night pizza night.
- Review your list and recognize what events and emotions are tied to the foods. Is it a coping mechanism when you were in college preparing for an exam? Is it what your mother gave you to make you feel better if you were sad? Was it Friday pizza specials that became a weekly ritual?
- Decide to work on only one of the emotional or event ties and began unraveling it by choosing a healthier food option. This allows a place holder while you work through disconnecting the feeling or event from that food. Eventually, you will become used to feeling upset, disappointed, and sad without having to reach for certain foods. The opportunity to disconnect is here!

- Remember, through every step you are working on shifting your mindset. The goal is to change your way of thinking by actively disconnecting from the pattern. From there, the emotional response can be handled in a more self-loving way.

PART II
Strategies for Winning

Finding Your *Why*

Dancing During Your Fight

Starting a Partnership

Moving to the Driver's Seat

Starting with a Transitional Approach

Being Ready for the Point of No Return

"We need to do a better job of putting ourselves higher on our own 'to do' list."

Michelle Obama

CHAPTER 6

FIND YOUR *WHY*

*"Your Why: What honors you?
What heals you?"*

WHAT IS YOUR ROOT REASON FOR MAKING CHANGES TO YOUR HEALTH?

When asked this question, many of my new clients tell me that their *Why* is losing weight, increasing energy, or building muscle. While these are reasonable goals, these common reasons are not rooted reasons that will keep most people on track during their weight-loss journey. It's easy to fall back into old routines when the reasons why we seek changes are more short-term fixes rather than a foundational mind shift that will lead to a long-term transformation.

To make sustainable changes, you must have a deeply embedded root *Why* reason centered around the questions, *"What honors you?"* and *"What heals you?"*

YOUR *WHY* MUST BE FOR YOU

Don't fall into the trap of making your *Why* statement about something or for someone else. Some examples are:
- I want to lose weight for my children.
- My significant other thinks I should lose weight.
- My doctor wants me to lose weight.

These indirect reasons are not the long-term drivers to keep you from reverting to unhealthy habits.

Instead, your *Why* reason(s) must be about you and no one else:
- I deserve to be a priority in my life.
- My needs are more important than others' wants.
- I'm worth it.
- I want my life to be lived to its fullest while feeling my best.
- I care enough about me to change me.

Using your *Why* as daily thoughts, affirmations, and declarations creates a solid foundation, empowering you to take ownership for long-term change. Repeating them throughout the day will also help keep you focused and on track during the day-to-day fight.

Your *Why* reason will establish a permanent base that is steadfast and sustainable. Your foundation will also be what you default to when times get frustrating or you think about giving up. You will always go back to your *Why*. Your *Why* will always link directly to you.

Being double rooted in your *Why* provides a foundation where growth and change can manifest. When you are double rooted in your *Why*, both your heart and mind are in sync. You are also embracing yourself and putting yourself first. Nothing is forced.

Remember, your foundation is about you alone. Once you have established your foundation, your *Why* reason can grow strong and can endure in the face of most obstacles.

🏆 HOW TO WIN! Creating Your *Why* Statement

If you are beginning to develop your *Why* statement, use these questions as guidance:
- How did you feel when you were at your best?
- How is your quality of life under your current living habits?
- Are you ready to make yourself a priority?
- What would it mean to look at your reflection and be proud of what you see?
- How badly do you desire to be the *you* that you deserve?

Also think about:
- What honors you? Consider who you choose to marry or where you decide to move your family. Your choices honor your deepest desires. In the same way, you can let your food choices honor you.
- What heals you? Consider where you go to hear encouragement or who you go to for advice to help you to grow and become a better you. Choose foods that heal you.

Then, take answers from these questions and fill in the following blanks:
1. At my best, I feel_____.
2. I envision my quality of life in 10 years to look like _____.
3. On _____ day, I am putting myself first.
4. I feel_____, see_____, and proud of _____ when I see my reflection in the mirror.
5. I desire_____ and deserve _____ for myself.

These are the foundations for your *Why*.

CHAPTER 7

ARE YOU FIGHTING A REPEAT WEIGHT-LOSS BATTLE?

"Look at losing weight like a bob and weave dance, not a fistfight in the ring."

STOP FIGHTING AND GET IN SYNC

Do you feel like you've been fighting your weight for your entire life? Have you been trying to force your body to change? Have you been determined to build muscle or lose fat weight and it didn't seem to work? Have you worked hard, to the point of exhaustion? Perhaps you're so exhausted that you've given up and feel as if you've lost the fight.

If you're like many of my clients, you feel that your body and the scale are the enemies. An enemy that always finds a way to win. And you are continually left feeling depleted and like you have lost the battle.

💬 MOLLY'S STORY

When Molly and I first met, she talked about all the diets she had been on that promised at least 20-pound weight loss. She lamented over the money wasted on diet plans, pre-packaged meal systems, and weight-loss products.

Molly found temporary weight-loss success, but in less than six months, she gained it all back. She desperately wanted to lose weight quickly and did anything to force her body to change.

Every diet venture turned into counting calories and making sacrificial changes to her foods to get the body she wanted. Those sacrifices involved declining date nights with her husband and girls' nights out with her friends so she could avoid situations tempting her to eat. She ate only vegetables and salads because they promised weight loss. She eliminated everything that had sugar to prevent weight gain. It was as if she was punishing herself because she didn't trust herself to go out and enjoy life, fearing that the food would win.

Every morning she determined her calorie intake based on what the scale said. If it tilted in her favor, she felt validated. If it didn't move, she was frustrated. If it went up, she dug in deeper to restrict and count calories.

During our conversations, I realized she had become bitter toward food and angry and judgmental toward herself.

She said, "I'm always fighting to change my body."

I asked, "How many times have you gone in the ring and thrown in the towel?"

Sighing, she replied, "I'm zero for ten."

Her energy was so low, and she sat exhausted and depleted.

Molly is like many people. Perhaps you can relate?

Molly and I worked together and identified areas that she found the most difficult. Then, we began developing solutions along with alternatives. Alternatives are necessary because everyone is different and what might work for one client might not work for another, especially the first time. I didn't want Molly to become more discouraged. It was time to raise her energy level and rebuild her self-confidence.

Molly had struggled with inconsistency in her meals because of her schedule and with taking time for exercise. She needed a plan that would work with her schedule. First, we created a routine of including portion-sized fruits and nuts as snacks to fit her busy workdays. She kept them close at hand, and this made it easier for her to eat consistently during the day. Second, she started walking three days a week for 30 minutes. Third, she listened to inspirational podcasts while walking, which kept her engaged and encouraged.

Molly won her fight by changing her approach. She added enjoyment to her routine and incorporated simple snacks into her schedule that worked well for her. She didn't feel stress, frustration, and bitterness, which allowed her to relax and get in sync. She naturally started losing weight, and the battle she fought in the past, no longer seemed like a fight.

As the weight began to fall off, Molly stopped punishing herself, began spending time with loved ones, and trusted herself to make healthy choices when she went out. Over time she reached and maintained her goal weight and went on to achieve other desired milestones because she believed in herself.

Remember, there is no honor or power in always fighting and losing. When you feel anxious, frustrated, or on edge because your body isn't changing fast enough, slow down and do the bob and weave dance.

I call this learning how to move with the punches instead of wasting your energy during the fight. That means learning how to be proactive in certain situations when you know a struggle is coming.

Here's an example: You are invited to a friend's party, and you know that there will be a buffet table weighted down with food and drinks. Don't go to the party ready to fight the temptation you know is coming. Approach the situation with a game plan and know how to avoid pitfalls.

Plan to eat ahead of time to avoid the temptation of filling your plate with what is available. Then, at the party, prepare a small sample plate. In advance, decide how you are going to balance your alcohol intake. Does that mean two drinks instead of four?

By having a plan and being proactive, you find steps and can anticipate your moves. Eventually, like any other skill, you become better prepared for facing any preconceived fight.

Remember that establishing new connections, building relationships, and making changes is a continual process. When you keep at it, you will be amazed at how the tiny steps add up to significant progress.

🏆 HOW TO WIN! Choosing Your Tune

Before professional bouts, fighters enter the ring to a song to "tune-up" the audience. It gets the crowd excited and ready for what's to come. Just like the professionals, we hype ourselves up (or down) every day without realizing how those tunes are affecting us. Often, our songs are justifications. What lyrics are in your head? *"I deserve to have this piece of cake." "I'll start next week after vacation." "I want to do what I want to do."* Does this sound familiar? If so, how's it working for you? What you sing or tell yourself can be damaging. If it's happening, it's time to change the station and listen to new lyrics.

Just think. What if you heard the following?
- I deserve more for myself than the extra calories from that piece of cake.
- I will start now, not tomorrow.
- I choose to do what's better for my health rather than what's tastier on my tongue.

If you need to change the lyrics in your head, do the following:
- Think about the negative talk you've heard yourself say in the past and begin telling yourself the opposite.
- Realize your thoughts create actions. To change your thoughts, you must change your actions.
- The moment a negative thought comes to mind, recognize it, stop it, and turn it into into positive thinking.
- Be aware of those around you who speak negatively. If necessary, find others who will encourage you through their positive energy and words.
- Stop creating unrealistic expectations. Create tangible goals that build on each other.
- Find your favorite mantras or words of affirmation and surround yourself with them.

Try it! The new lyrics may even ignite other aspects of your life!

🏆 HOW TO WIN! Changing Your Internal Conversation

Just because you chose to eat a slice of pie over a bowl of fruit doesn't mean you are bad or being bad. The moment you call yourself bad, it influences other choices with negative consequences. The next step could quickly turn into being "bad" the entire night.

Tell yourself you could have made a better choice, recognizing that you chose the pie, and be intentional in choosing differently next time.

Judgment works both ways. Think about the times when you claimed to have been "good" all day. You put unnecessary/undue pressure on yourself to stay "good." This thought pattern is like walking on ice because if you slip and make one mistake, you immediately go back to the "bad me" thinking.

Change your thoughts and internal conversation to acknowledging that you are practicing and making progress consistently and choosing better choices that align with the goals you are setting for yourself. Practicing builds the foundation for success, as lasting change never happens immediately.

Do you have a hard time changing your internal conversation? Tell – and promise – yourself the following:
- I must be patient with myself.
- I will not strive for perfection but reach for progress.
- When I strive for 100%, I can set myself up for failure. I will work on consistently being in the 85% club.
- I express self-love by every healthy choice I make, and that is better for my well-being.
- I care about my body, my life, and my future enough to make food healthy choices.
- My past actions do not define my present and future.
- I will drown out negative thoughts with words of empowerment.
- I determine who I am to become.

CHAPTER 8

FOOD WEARS MANY HATS, BUT WHICH HAT IT WEARS IS UP TO YOU

"Make a change and breathe. Make another change and breathe. Realize that if we are not connected to ourselves, we are subject to the power we have given away."

Food is a chameleon that wears many hats and has many names. Many times, we give it titles that provide us with a false sense of security. It has worn the hat of a savior, our go-to, a comforter, our reward – and many more!

And food usually doesn't live up to the names we give it. When we indulge, we are often left feeling empty. The hats we assign to our food choices essentially become a place holder for the emotions or events we are not ready to face. Because of that, we give up our power to those foods.

Have you ever gone to a dinner party and swore you had to stay away from the dessert table? Why? Because if you get too close, you will lose your control (power). Or have you looked at a plate of food and thought, *"I can't have that!"*

If so, you're giving food reign over your ability to make decisions for yourself.

What hats have you given food in your life? Maybe the following sound familiar:
- My reward (because I deserve it)
- My relief (when you're overwhelmed)
- My routine (when chaos happens)
- My familiar friend (when you're lonely)
- My time-filler (when you're bored)
- My comforter (when you're anxious)
- My soother (when you're upset)
- My happiness (when you're sad or already happy)

Your thoughts, as well as your words, determine your interpretation of food. When you think, *"I can't,"* you are saying something is stronger than you. You are saying you are weak in comparison.

It's time to stop the revolving door that keeps perpetuating a negative cycle. It's time to stop giving food permission to define who you are. Strip foods of its stars and take its power away. Instead, position yourself in the seat of power by changing your narrative.

Change, *"I can't have that"* to *"I am choosing not to have that right now."* Change *"I can't be around certain foods"* to *"I decide what I will have. Food doesn't decide for me."*

While you're at it, change hats and acknowledge that while food may have been an adversary in the past, you want it to be a partner moving forward. Give food the hats of healer, lifeline, fuel, and vitality. Then go about choosing healthy food options, which are in alignment with self-care.

TAKE A BREATH BETWEEN ROUNDS

Look at the steps leading to lasting change like taking a breath. Whenever you are about to face something new or challenging, you have always been taught to take a deep breath. Take a deep breath to prepare yourself to slow down and understand you are learning a methodical dance that will help you win the fight. When you take a breath, you can focus, you can calm yourself, and you can think more clearly.

Breathing also means understanding you are human, and you will make mistakes. That doesn't mean you are losing. It means you are in tune and aligning yourself to living into this change of eating, and that takes time.

A PARTNERSHIP WITH HEALTHY FOOD STARTS HERE
Affirm and commit to choosing food that benefits your body. **See healing and nutrition as companions who help your body and empower you to want the best choices.** This way of thinking is the beginning of the mental shift you began to experience when seeing food as a partner. It also opens a different way of interacting with what you consume. You start to change your language to words of positivity and strength behind your words.

Take your control back by changing *"I can't"* to *"I choose."* Choosing internally, from a place of awareness rather than hunger or comfort, is where your power lies.

Here's what an internal conversation sounds like: *"I may want that piece of pie, but I am choosing this bowl of fruit because it's best for my health."*

When you establish that you are running the show, you become the victor instead of succumbing to the unhealthy food adversary.

HOW TO WIN!
The Power of Personal Proclamations

When you proclaim your position, it comes from a place of wanting better for yourself. It comes from the heart and proclaiming it means you believe it. You believe yourself.

Make these proclamations to yourself:
- I will try to be aware of my thoughts, feelings, and emotions.
- I choose to care for my needs by prioritizing what's most important *now* rather than ignoring, procrastinating, or rationalizing.
- I am working on food and its connection to me. As a result, I am moving forward.
- I am my best partner! My awareness makes me a better partner to myself.

CHAPTER 9

YOU ARE THE DRIVER IN CHARGE

"Invest in yourself by deciding it's all about your self-care first and be okay with that. Move to the driver's seat, take off, and reclaim your vitality!"

How do you feel about yourself, and where do you prioritize your health? Are you often last on the totem pole, taking the left-over time, using the last vapors of energy, or dragging along on the "give it a try" spectrum? You may feel it's more important to care for those you love and never address your own needs. Perhaps you feel guilty if you take time to care for yourself?

The people who know you well know the buttons to push to make you "feel" guilty or to do what's in their best interests (contradicting yours at times). You are as important as the people you love. And let's face it, what would their quality of life be if you were not around? Often, we disregard our feelings or needs by making excuses without realizing we are doing so. That's no way to live.

When you are in the driver's seat, you are responsible for your thoughts, feelings, emotions, activities, and the way you react to life's occurrences.

SELF-SACRIFICING TRANSLATES INTO LACK OF SELF-WORTH

To be clear, choosing to put yourself first does not mean your care for others is less important. Let go of self-sacrificing by prioritizing what's most important that day. And when something comes up, which it will, re-prioritize and remind yourself that you can manage change. When things fall apart, fix what you can. Also, learn from each situation and mistake, and then move on instead of feeling down, defeated, or guilty.

I know many times that's easier said than done.

Too often, especially for caregivers and parents, most of our guilt is self-imposed because we tend to internalize problems and issues. The opposite can also be true if we are faced with external conflicts and take all the responsibility and bear the negative energy from others. When faced with these internal and external forces, we get a double whammy. It's easy, almost natural, to soak up our guilt and the guilt we allow others to make us feel. Then, we are down for the count, tired, and unable to focus on self-care.

I like to use the analogy of the back-seat driver. If you are a parent, a caregiver, or a person who cares about others more than yourself, then you know what it feels like to sit in the back seat. You aren't in control of the vehicle. Others dictate your actions.

If you had to be at work in thirty minutes, would you give your car keys to a random stranger on the way to the job and offer them a joy ride, as long as you could sit in the back seat of your vehicle, on the way to the building? Of course not! You would not allow it to happen! When we take on too much, and then feel guilty or less-than because we can't keep up, that's what we're doing. We are letting something or someone else drive.

💬 DOUG'S, THE SUPER DAD'S, STORY

Doug has four small children. When he wakes in the morning, his first thought is to make sure they have a substantial breakfast, so they are prepared for the day. Even though his kids eat a nutritious breakfast, every morning Doug finds himself skipping breakfast, racing to grab a cup of coffee, and running out of the door to work.

By not taking the time to slow down and have a good breakfast, he neglects to care for himself.

The result? Self-sabotage.

Because he didn't supply his body with the nutrients it deserves and needs, he felt tired, irritated, and depleted during the day. He was unable to give 100% because he didn't have it to give.

This routine was a repeating pattern. And over time, Doug eventually became desensitized to the unhealthy habit.

After so many rounds of the same scenario, Doug realized this is not the way to live, and he deserved better.

🏆 HOW TO WIN! Move to the Driver's Seat

Deciding to carve out time for yourself puts you in the driver's seat, feeds your family, and doesn't take away from your role as caregiver or self-caregiver. Even if you choose to do this once a week, it's a start! You have to start somewhere to begin restoring your energy, which allows you to operate at full capacity.

Do you struggle in the mornings? Consider following the steps below to carve out some extra time that will give you energy and focus:
- Wake up 15 minutes early to prepare a breakfast that takes 5 minutes to make.
- Take 10 minutes to eat and enjoy a peaceful cup of coffee. Gather your thoughts and prepare for your day.

Because you made time for yourself first, an extra 15 minutes can go a long way to helping you feel better. And you will be able to handle issues now that you are more equipped to deal with the day.

Let's face it. After a long day when it's time to eat dinner, you may not have the energy to cook. It may be tempting to stop at a fast-food restaurant and pick up something. Instead, try the following:
- Choose a nearby grocery store.
- Shop for fresh, prepared food, grab it, and go. It's convenient and healthier.
- Take advantage of food and grocery delivery services.
- Pre-order your healthy meals from health-conscious restaurants.

By following these simple steps, you can reach the end of the day, feeling more in control and successful. Another reward is feeling better physically.

Congratulations! This is how it feels to win every day!

CHAPTER 10

BUILDING BETTER CONFIDENCE

*"When you know more,
you can do better."*

Many times, we don't experience success because we don't know where to start, where to go, or who to believe. Also, we might not have the necessary knowledge to move forward. When our knowledge is limited, we are limited.

Have you heard the Chinese proverb, *"Give a man a fish, and you feed him for a day but teach a man to fish, and you feed him for a lifetime."*? This saying explains that it's better to teach someone to do something rather than to do it for them. By doing so, you equip them with confidence to take care of themselves.

It's time to learn how to fish!

We live in a society where we depend on a program or system telling us how to eat, how to lose weight, or how to be healthier without teaching us how to do it for ourselves. This approach skews your ability to incorporate healthy foods into your unique life dynamics.

In the past, you may have found yourself following a system that assigned points to various foods. You go for it because it's easy and it gives you rules. However, you only learn how to count and keep tabs. But you don't fully understand what's going on or why the rules are there.

For example, if you eat an egg-white omelet only because you're following the rules of a plan, you don't learn about its benefits. This approach is limiting and won't last.

On the other hand, think about how you feel about the omelet when you understand its benefits:
- A good option for weight loss
- A fat-free, low cholesterol protein source

Furthermore, even though you lose some of the nutrients and vitamins from the yolk, you can add other nutrients by adding veggies to your omelet. When you have this information, you begin to connect the dots and are more likely to continue preparing and eating the omelet.

CONFIDENCE MAKES CHANGE HAPPEN

When facing the prospect of significant change, it can be overwhelming and seemingly impossible at times, especially when it comes to understanding food and what approach is best for you.

I hear many people say, *"I don't want to think about it."* I interpret that as, *"I don't want to take the time to learn my body and how it responds to food."* I get that change can be difficult and burdensome, and the process can seem impossible when you have a long list of other life commitments. However, to be successful, you must invest the time and effort in you.

When building confidence, you must want to know more than just a calorie count, a point system, or a macro percentage. Failure often happens when you don't start at the beginning and take the necessary steps for understanding food and its effect on your body. Instead of moving forward, you fall back and lose confidence.

Start by learning about nutrition and what syncs with your life dynamics. A simplistic approach is often best and will help you transition. **Take your time with measured steps, which is better than tackling the whole subject at one time.**

I know you want to become a quick expert but think about how long it takes to build self-confidence, assurance, and mastery in any area of life. It involves time, patience, determination, education, and experience. Mechanics may start tinkering in the garage. Hairstylists might begin practicing in the mirror. Future doctors may start with hopes and dreams as first graders before graduating from medical school and passing certification exams.

No one steps out and becomes proficient in their skills overnight. They must learn the basics and what they need to equip themselves best.

🏆 HOW TO WIN! Start with a Transitional Approach

Transitional change is a winning approach to meeting your health and body goals. Knowing and understanding what works for your body creates desired results. As a dietitian, I say, *"Add a little, and subtract a little over time and be intentional with learning as you go."*

What does transitional change look like when it comes to making the right food choices? Let's look at vegetables and fried foods, for example. We all know vegetables are essential to our health, but they can be the hardest food group to eat daily. If getting enough vegetables during the day is one of your challenges, try to start adding (or transitioning) veggies to your major meals first. It doesn't have to be a lot.

Maybe fried foods are your weakness. Attempt to subtract them sometimes from your meals. I am not saying to disassociate yourself from fried foods. Just have them less.

Then, while you are in the transitional stage of adding vegetables (slowly) and subtracting fried foods (gradually) take time to learn about the benefits of vegetables. I stress slowly and gradually because transitions and building knowledge take time.

Then, incorporate watching 3-minute videos or reading short articles about interesting vegetables and how to prepare them, focusing on benefits. You will find plenty of room for variety and exploration.

By learning in small bites, you will eventually add more vegetables to your meals, which leads to more vegetables on every plate. You'll be eating vegetables because of what you are learning, not because of the rules. And you are choosing to minimize your fried foods, rather than forcing yourself to take away fried foods. The more you learn, the more confidence you will have.

CHAPTER 11
THE POINT OF NO RETURN

"In tears she couldn't believe the scale. Forty-three pounds heavier since the divorce was filed, less than three months ago. At that moment, she wanted to crawl in her bed and eat some rocky road ice cream."

THE POINT OF NO RETURN BATTLE

The point of no return is the moment when you are face to face with your adversary (food), and you are caught in an emotional trance. You know you are not willing to turn the other direction and say no. You are going to embrace that adversary and enjoy every single second of the encounter.

There's nothing stronger than the desire to want the extra piece of cake or a second serving of your favorite pasta dish. All rationale, all self-proclamations, and all will power have dissolved, and there is only one direction you are going. Towards that food!

The moment of no return is such a strong connection that you can't think of anything else, and nothing will satisfy the urge. You can't get past the feeling until that embrace, that encounter, that consumption of that thing happens.

RECOGNIZING THE POINT OF NO RETURN

Have you ever said, *"Next time, I'll pass,"* or *"It's the weekend, so I can loosen up and have a second helping"*? We've all experienced these predicaments and have given in to our deep-felt need to feed. We "just do it" and most times we make our justifications, giving in to our indulgences no matter the cost. However, these actions can become a repeated cycle, giving our adversary (food) every chance to beat us.

Yes, I said, beat! The issue is, you may not have even known you were in a fight. Comfort foods often dull the senses and make you feel better for those five seconds of pleasure, sacrificing your body for your tongue's delight.

But when you take a step back and think about it, the consequences of giving in to the craving is not worth it. The guilt and the weight that builds up over time makes it more challenging to break the cycle and free yourself from the habit of feeding the sensation. The results can be agonizing and long term.

FIGHTING THE POINT OF NO RETURN
Even though it may seem that you are always in a losing battle, you can win and beat the adversary. However, it takes the presence of mind, heart, and caring enough to desire the victory.

You must work to battle the cravings, the emotions, and overcoming the desires and desperations of the tongue and whatever may have been driving you toward that food/those experiences.

Awareness and an action plan will build your confidence, like the examples below can prepare you for the fight when the adversary shows up in the ring.
- Start by visualizing what you are going to do when confronted by the challenge. Winging it never works!
- Remember, each encounter is an opportunity to learn and prepare for the next round.
- Keep in mind practice makes progress, not perfect. The more you stick to your plan, the better – and more agile – you will become at playing offense.
- Know that life will continue to throw challenges in your path.

WINNING FEELS GOOD

We all face times when we are stuck between what we want for ourselves and what we want in those bags of chips! The point of no return is a trap we can't escape.

But imagine stepping into the winner's circle and think about the feeling you will have as you get stronger in finding ways to evade vulnerable moments. In the beginning, it may feel like the hardest struggle. But if you genuinely want to taste victory over the temptations of food, you will learn to recognize what foods, situations, and feelings make you exposed to food temptation.

You deserve winning moments, and as you become stronger, you will have more of those moments. Nothing feels better than to know you are winning the food fight. You are a champion, and your choices will confirm that every time you choose to take power away from foods.

🏆 HOW TO WIN!
Arming Yourself Against the Point of No Return

Before we declare victory, we must identify what we're doing and what we're not doing. In other words, we must be actively engaged with ourselves, not blindly following our emotions or desiring what tastes good on our tongues.

Consider the following strategies for preparing yourself for food challenges:

- **Stop at the Store.** We are surrounded by tempting food many times because it's in the house and close at hand. If there are foods impossible to ignore when they are in your cabinet, pantry, or refrigerator, leave them in the aisle at the grocery store. Keep walking and prevent "the point of no return" moment.

- **Pause to Inspect Ahead.** If you know there is a party coming up Friday night and there are bound to be your favorite desserts there, create a mental game plan about how the scenario will play out. Decide before you go if you are going to bypass the desserts or pick one out of the spread and find balance in that. You must think ahead because if you don't, there will be a point of return moment.
- **Handle the Workplace Snack Table.** Every workplace has a snack spot where co-workers bring donuts or leftover cake from their kid's birthday party. When it's unexpected, what do you do? One solution is to have prepared snacks at your desk. Pack your favorite granola bars or trail mix, so you have something to satisfy your sweet tooth. This strategy will also help you control portion sizes and ease the cravings that many experience from smelling that chocolate cake in the breakroom. I guarantee you will feel better about your choice versus being within the trance of the point of no return.

Remember, you can be bold, confident, and victorious in a battle when you know what you are fighting and know how to fight.

PART III
Preparing for Challenges

Recognizing Patterns

Learning Associations and Attachments

Preparing for the Unexpected

"If you are proactive, you focus on preparing. If you are reactive, you end up focusing in repairing."

John C. Maxwell

CHAPTER 12
PATTERNS, PATTERNS, PATTERNS!

"Patterns are a particular way in which something is done or organized, or in which something happens, according to the Cambridge Dictionary. However, certain patterns undermine our ability to change results and reach our goals."

Patterns are embedded actions and reactions you may find yourself doing almost unconsciously. When you stop to think about it, you can identify patterns in many areas of your life that you might not otherwise recognize because they are automatic. For example, every morning you wake up, drink a cup of coffee, take a shower, then watch TV while getting ready. Perhaps on Wednesday evenings, your pattern is watching your favorite TV show, sifting through the news, and getting the kids ready for bed. Or on a Sunday afternoon, you catch up on housework, get in a good read, and go to the local ice cream shop.

There is power in these patterns. Because they are embedded in our routine, breaking and re-programming patterns can seem like a daunting task. Even though existing patterns are often difficult to change or stop, people usually have an easy time falling into the rhythm of a new routine.

How do we address breaking food patterns? The first step is recognizing how food patterns are connected to rituals.

FOOD PATTERNS AND RITUALS

If every evening on your way home from work you snack on chips or a candy bar, you develop a habit in the car. Eventually, without thinking about it, that snack becomes your evening ritual, a way to unwind after a hard day of work. This pattern becomes a habit connected to your physical and mental process of leaving work and coming home. If you were to forget your snack, you might feel something is absent. Are you missing the snack, or are you missing the habit of eating in the car? You may not realize you have become stuck in a pattern of eating out of habit and when you may not be hungry.

Honestly, some patterns are challenging to break because they are deeply embedded acts that provide safety and familiarity.

BREAKING PATTERNS AND HABITS

To break a pattern requires separating who you are from the established habit/pattern. The temptation may be to resist the change or to revert to the pattern because it's comfortable.

Remember, that choosing discomfort to break a habit and achieve your goal takes effort, but that's the way to overcome what's not working for you.

It's possible to keep the routine but change the pattern, replacing it with something better that is in alignment with your goals.

For example, if snacking on crunchy kettle chips while driving home from work in rush hour traffic is your thing, okay. But you've gained 10 pounds in the past three months since you started commuting, and you may not be satisfied with those results. Perhaps it's time to skip the chips? Then it's time to repattern.

Think about the simplicity of replacing the chips with a healthier choice like pretzels or fruit.

Repatterning allows the pattern of snacking to continue. Simply change what you decide to snack on. You may still have a taste for chips during your evening commute but pausing for a minute and acknowledging the drivetime ritual will allow you to rethink your choices.

> **🏆 HOW TO WIN!**
> **Skip the Chips and Repattern Your Rituals**

There are many ways to win the repatterning battle, and it's not always about eliminating food options. Consider the following strategies for choosing healthier choices:
- **Grocery store cookies.** If you are a fan of the serve-yourself cookies in the bakery cookie case, grab one cookie instead of three and keep going.
- **Vending machines.** Rather than debating which candy bar to choose, go for the granola or trail mix. You will still get the sweetness but in a healthier way.
- **Sporting events.** When you are at the baseball game (or any other sporting event), and the snack guys make their rounds, grab the popcorn or peanuts. Then, remind yourself the game will be great without the extra calories from the nachos and hotdogs.
- **Fast-food restaurants.** In today's busy world when time is at a premium, fast-food restaurants often save us time. Scope out the ones that offer healthier options and go for the grilled chicken sandwich, skipping the fries or opting for a side of fruit.
- **Movie theaters.** If you're like most moviegoers, a film on the big screen isn't complete without nachos, popcorn, and a soda. To avoid this pitfall, bring snacks from home or choose to share a small popcorn with your date.
- **Home alone.** The perfect storm has hit. You are upset, your favorite movie is on, and you are alone this weekend. Instead of buying a gallon of ice cream, downsize to a personal size carton and try one with lower sugar. Remember, you won't feel good after emptying the larger tub.

- **Holidays.** It's the holiday, and your mom made her famous chocolate cake. Don't skip it! Decide to have a smaller-sized sample piece and remember not to create an excuse about wanting a second serving. Focus on enjoying time with family, not calories.

CHAPTER 13

ASSOCIATIONS AND ATTACHMENTS

"Most holidays, celebrations, and social events are intentionally created around food, and we frequently overindulge."

We often associate foods with certain occurrences in our lives without thinking about it. These associations often lead to unintentional eating that can create unfavorable results.

RECOGNIZING UNHEALTHY ASSOCIATIONS AND ATTACHMENTS

Think about when you find yourself having random cravings. Are they associated with a time, an event, or a scenario? Here are a few instances:

- When you go to the movies, you immediately crave popcorn.
- When you go to a baseball game, you make a point to grab a hot dog and soda.
- When you feel anxious, you go for the cookies.
- When you're sad, you reach for ice cream.
- When you're at a birthday party or wedding, you can't wait to eat the cake!

Any other time, these specific foods are not necessarily on your radar. You are less likely to be interested in a hot dog, soda, or cookie on a random occasion.

These cravings arise because we associate foods with events and how we feel. Food is connected to both positive and negative events. You may have been rewarded for having good grades or winning a game during your childhood. For example, if your mom baked brownies every time your team won, the connection to the reward is the enjoyment of eating the brownies. So, every time you think brownies, you see it as a reward.

Recognizing that you want brownies after an achievement or that you get cravings for pizza on Friday nights is likely about your past experiences and attachments to these items.

Let's be clear. All associations aren't always positive. When you get anxious or upset and feel like cookies are magically calling your name, you indulge, as if eating them will make it all better. Could it have been that as a child, your mom gave you cookies to make you feel better? Perhaps eating is not about the cookies but perceiving them as the remedy or companion to your problem? After the indulgence, do they fill the void? Likely not. They only reinforce a cycle of continued association.

Emotions play an influential role in your relationship with food, whether you realize it or not. I like to think of our connection to food and emotions like a ball and chain. Certain foods and the feelings you associate with them are tied together and stay attached to your ankle, pulling you back and holding you down. If you are feeling bad, food is there. If you are feeling good, food is there. If you are feeling anxious, food is there. If you are bored, food is there. Food is here, there, and everywhere. Do you see the ball and chain?

You may have gone your entire life not understanding why you have been attached to certain foods. Now that you *know* about those attachments, you can unravel the connections and make different choices.

BREAKING THE ASSOCIATION AND ATTACHMENT CYCLE

Many people are emotional eaters and don't realize it. However, many of my clients do recognize it and proclaim, *"I'm an emotional eater, and I know it."* Acknowledgment is good; however, don't permit yourself to continue to live that way.

How do we break the cycle? After you recognize the associations and attachments, you must disconnect from them.

Easier said than done, right?

But you can break the ball and chain by detaching your emotions from food. Separating your feelings can be time consuming and takes consistent effort. Decide to loosen one chain link at a time. This can mean letting go of the soda, start purchasing bite-size candy bars instead of the larger versions, or buying single-size packs of nuts instead of a larger jar.

You can pick which link you work on first and then keep disconnecting.

Here's another way to think about this: If you are the one who craves pizza every Friday night, try changing what you eat when Friday night comes. This simple decision will be the first step in creating an intentional separation from needing to have pizza on Friday nights. You are essentially taking away the power of the pizza in your life. If you must, try having pizza on a different night to lessen the association with Friday intentionally.

You can also create different associations when dealing with difficult emotions, rather than staying attached to eating food that won't solve your issues.

If you reach for cookies when you feel anxious or upset, stop to recognize and evaluate how you feel at this moment and how you want to feel in the next hour.

When you recognize that your emotions are driving you to crave or consume food at a specific time, pause and ask yourself if food is the answer or if something else needs to be addressed. I guarantee that most of the time, food isn't the answer.

You always have a choice. You can decide to waffle and stay with your current mindset that doesn't change the problem, or you can choose to control your decisions. Having the courage to control your choices can be intimidating. But recognize that this conversation is not about the cookies. Instead, it's about managing your emotions, acknowledging associations, and choosing not to be attached to eating for perceived comfort. When you work through attachments this way, you begin to reclaim your power.

Self-awareness and being intentional about why you're making certain choices break the cycle of event-associated attachments.

HANDLING CHALLENGES AND STRESS

Challenges and stress are common. Unfortunately, you may not be able to "fix" what's causing the stress. But you can control how you decide to deal with it. It takes standing still during the chaos. It takes refusing to relive past cycles.

When faced with events or occurrences that may have resulted in unintentional eating in the past, take a different approach. Identify if the reaction is circumstantial or emotional then make an intentional choice to respond. If you're tempted to eat the brownie only for comfort, choose differently. Deal with the emotions first/separately. However, if the brownie is actually what you want (independently), don't deny yourself.

Remember, our goal is to detach from attachments that are not in line with our goals. As you continue to *practice* disconnecting, eventually ties will be released.

🏆 HOW TO WIN!
Mindset Change for New Associations

Breaking the chain is hard, especially when reverting to old habits is easy; however, it's a process worth going through. To disassociate yourself from the current cycle, you must first change your mindset. Think about the following:
- Acknowledge that you have an emotional attachment to food.
- Recognize what events repetitively trigger specific food cravings. Is it at night? On a road trip? When watching your favorite TV show? When your best friend comes for a visit? At every birthday party? Stop to think about how this played out last time and how you felt right afterward.
- Ask yourself, *"Is it worth it?" "Will it take me back into the same emotional spiral?" "How can I choose something different this time?" "Is this in line with what I want for myself?"*
- Make a conscious effort to make unemotional healthier food choices to create a new association. Instead of grabbing the chips and dip, grab the chips and salsa. Swap the big bowl of ice cream for an individual low-fat ice cream bar. Instead of making it a taco night, make it a taco salad night. Decide the candy bar isn't the answer, but a small bag of trail mix may do the trick!
- Know that change – and you – are worth the effort.

A mind shift begins with being mentally aware and recognizing associations. Change comes second. Once you know your triggers, you can establish new patterns aligned with your goals. Through repetition, these new habits will become your new normal.

CHAPTER 14

THINGS POP UP! WHAT ARE YOU GOING TO DO?

"Getting through circumstances and making healthy choices consistently takes practice. You can do it when you don't give up on yourself!"

When you decide to develop healthier eating habits, you might expect that that life will be smooth without any unforeseen interruptions. But you can't always know – and plan for – the obstacles on the horizon.

If you are like many others, you may push new habits to the side when unexpected circumstances arise to better focus on the unexpected problem at hand. Also, you may feel overwhelmed and want to give in only to start over after things settle down.

Spoiler alert! Life is about change, unexpected events, unhappy experiences, and celebratory moments. There will be times when distractions will discombobulate you. And your emotions will always be connected to the changes. Furthermore, when you add food to the mix, you may find it challenging to maintain the eating habits you vowed you would keep.

Even though you may feel defeated and exhausted, the key is to persevere through these challenges. If you do, you will keep moving forward toward your goals. Remember that if you continuously are on the start-stop yo-yo whenever there's a holiday, vacation, or stress-related event, you will never win the final round.

THE DERAILING POWER OF SELF-SABOTAGE

Self-sabotage is one of the surest things that keeps us off track. It usually stems from negative experiences in the past. Then, when similar experiences return, you hear that familiar voice inside your head say, *"I didn't do it. I couldn't do it. I can't do it now."*

But your internal voice doesn't have to be true.

If you think about the times when you didn't accomplish your goals, or you overindulged in something, it was likely because a circumstance unexpectedly popped up.

Maybe you had to work later than planned, which led to you skipping dinner and feeling overwhelmed because you found yourself with no prepared food. Or maybe at the last minute, you get a stressful phone call that brought back feelings you thought were resolved.

What do you when you want food in these situations when making healthier choices feels impossible? In these moments, you may feel like it's easier to give up or give in.

If you're like many people, you will forget every new goal you had and reach for food that's easy and quick. Most of the time, that means reverting to your former habits and self-defeating behaviors.

However, before you throw your hands up in defeat, realize whatever caused the stress was not anything you could have avoided, or what you can control. Even though events may affect you, it's up to you as to how you will react.

LOOK FOR OPPORTUNITIES IN THE UNEXPECTED

Every action you choose originates from the way you process events. If it is inevitable that things are going to pop up, decide these will be opportunities to approach events differently this time around. If you look to expect the unexpected, you will be able to see opportunity instead of feeling anger and frustration.

When you recognize that something outside of your control is influencing you, it gives you the power to make a different choice. Starting there, you can create new patterns, habits, associations, and plans leading to better self-care.

Taking care of yourself means putting yourself first no matter what pops up. Instead of putting yourself to the side when situations arise, think about how this may affect you, and then do what's in your best interest. When you continue to make healthy choices, no matter what happens, consistency becomes your everyday practice and your new normal.

💬 RICK'S STORY

When I met Rick, he said that he was always good at starting a healthy diet, but his problem was not sticking with it beyond two weeks. He was determined to follow his new program. Even though he was determined, Rick found out that he had to leave town unexpectedly for business, and that his family was making a last-minute weekend visit.

He was overwhelmed with thoughts of how to maintain a healthy lifestyle while navigating airports, holed up at long business meetings, and entertaining potential clients for dinner.

At that moment, Rick's easiest decision was to ignore his new goals. However, during this unpredictable moment, he recognized trips like this are part of his career, and he would have to learn what to do. Even though it was challenging to pack his snacks and look up restaurants in the area that fit his needs, he felt good about how he handled it afterward. He realized that to build consistency, he had to look at this "challenge" as an "opportunity" instead.

The real challenge occurred when his family came to town, and he had to scramble to make sure they were comfortable, and they had things to do. His immediate instinct was to drop everything to accommodate his family, but he then took a moment and realized this was a chance to put his needs first.

Instead of taking them to a baseball game, he took them to the zoo where healthy food choices were more prominent. Then, he decided to grill at home instead of eating out, so he had more control over the food choices.

It took a different way of thinking and more advanced planning to work through these unexpected events. But Rick knew if he wanted to stop the yo-yo cycle, he would have to be ready to work through life's challenges.

🏆 HOW TO WIN! Beating Unpredictability

How many times have you set a "perfect" plan in place for it to collapse? You planned to have breakfast and were ready to prepare it when you got a call saying you were needed "now"! Or you woke up late and the kids have to be at school in exactly 10 minutes!

Your reaction is to put off what you can (your breakfast) to get where you are needed, so you say, *"I don't have time to eat this morning. I will grab something after the meeting."*

Then, the meeting went thirty minutes longer than expected, and now you only have 15 minutes for lunch. You didn't bring a lunch. The lines in the cafeteria are way too long. Your next meeting is about to begin. So, you grab a quick snack from the closest vending machine to "hold you over." By that afternoon, you are exhausted physically and mentally and drink a soda in the car.

Once you are back home feeling stressed and hungry, you overeat and feel like a failure. You feel discouraged and disappointed, thinking, *"It is impossible to make the necessary changes in my life! I can't control this unpredictability!"*

Since you can't beat unpredictability, you must plan for it. Think about the following quick tips:
- Make lunch out of last night's leftovers. It takes less than 5 minutes to pack your lunch after dinner, especially if you pack before putting the rest of the food in a separate container.
- Have quick breakfast foods on hand (Greek yogurt cups, hardboiled eggs, or a piece of fruit).
- Add healthy snacks in your bag, briefcase, desk, or your car (nuts, a mini bag of pretzels, or a granola bar).
- Beating unpredictability also means recognizing outside influences that trigger emotions that might throw you off track. Be aware of others around you and your environment:
- Do they question or encourage you?
- Do they relentlessly offer you treats, or do they ask you first what you prefer?
- Do they make smug comments, or do they commend you for making healthy choices?
- Are you in a place where healthy options are around?
- Do you have accessibility to local markets and grocery stores?
- Do you actively seek restaurants with healthier menus?

- Do you intentionally surround yourself with positive energy?
- Do you explore ways to grow (i.e., podcasts, support groups, radio, and TV programs)?
- Do you spend your free time reading literature that enriches you?

Then, answer the following questions to formulate a plan and keep your goals in sight.

1. What/who are your external influencers?

   _____

   _____

2. How do they affect you?

   _____

   _____

3. What are ways you can address or avoid the negative influences?

   _____

   _____

4. What are the ways you can change, modify, and create positive influences?

   _____

   _____

5. What does it mean to *you* by creating new patterns and choices?

   _____

   _____

Remember, it isn't easy putting yourself first, and it's natural to feel uncomfortable when new changes are taking root. However, when you put yourself first, you are making yourself a priority.

PART IV
Know Your Allies and Opponents

Drinking Water

Knocking Out Empty Calories

Avoiding Preservatives

Eating for Your Metabolism

Facing Temptations

"Knowledge is a treasure, but practice is the key to it."

Lao Tzu

CHAPTER 15

YOU NEED WATER

"Water is your body's lifeline. When you give your body good hydration, it can do more."

Water is your body's habitat and makes up 66% of your body. Every system, muscle, tissue, and cell in your body needs water to function correctly.

When you don't give your body the hydration it needs, your immune system, among other organs and systems, is compromised. You stunt your body's ability to develop and heal when you don't hydrate. And, if you're like most people, you don't drink enough water.

BENEFITS OF DRINKING WATER

Water does more than quench your thirst. It also cleanses your body, helping to rid itself of toxins, and digests food. It increases brain power, provides energy, and breaks down and mobilizes fat molecules.

When you drink water, the benefits seem endless:
- Increases brain power and provides energy
- Promotes healthy weight management and weight loss
- Flushes out toxins
- Improves your complexion
- Maintains regularity
- Boosts immune system
- Prevents headaches
- Prevents cramps and injuries

HOW MUCH WATER SHOULD YOU DRINK?

Staying hydrated is essential. While many people stress the importance of drinking at least eight 8-ounce glasses of water a day, there's no cookie cutter rule because some people may need more.

How much water you should drink depends on your weight, how active you are, and how much you sweat. Of course, you should always drink water when you are thirsty.

On average, women should have around 11 cups of water a day (or 88 ounces) while men need slightly more at approximately 16 cups of water a day (or 128 ounces). These numbers may seem impossible, but keep in mind that you get about 20% of your daily water from the food that you eat.

🏆 HOW TO WIN! Creating a Hydration Action Plan

If you find it hard to drink enough water every day, try some of these suggestions:
- Make water interesting. Try infusing it with fruit for a fresh burst of flavor.
- Keep an insulated water bottle filled with ice water at your nightstand, so you drink first thing in the morning.
- Drink water during breakfast, lunch, and dinner, and with all your snacks.
- Purchase carbonated water to give yourself variety.
- Swap water for other favorite beverages or drink water along with other beverages.
- Fill and refrigerate water bottles, so you can quickly grab cold water when you leave home.
- Download a water intake app to get reminders (we all forget!).
- Purchase water bottles that have markings. These are fun!
- Carry a water bottle with you all the time. Think of it as an additional limb.

CHAPTER 16

KNOCK OUT EMPTY CALORIE OPTIONS

"When we feed our body, we don't realize we are feeding our brain first!"

Did you know that your brain is 2% of your body weight, yet it utilizes 20% of the nutrients you eat? When we starve ourselves or eat foods without nutrient value, we take away our ability to think clearly.

Eat regularly for your body and your mind. If nothing else, take time to feed your brain!

DOUGHNUTS OR PEANUTS

A handful of peanuts and a single doughnut carry equal amounts of fat calories. The difference is that nuts contain "healthy" fats. On the other hand, doughnuts give calories without nutrients, which means "unhealthy" fats.

Whenever possible, choose foods that are nutrient-dense over those that are calorie-dense. In this case, select the peanuts with the "healthy" fats that provide nutrients and will fuel your body and mind.

FUEL INSTEAD OF FATIGUE

Your relationship with food can support you in achieving your ultimate goals in life, whatever they may be. Without going into a scientific tirade, the food/nutrition you choose can fuel or fatigue your body.

Often overlooked, we tend to take food for granted, consuming what may taste good or what may seem the quickest or easiest at the moment. We also tend to ignore the impact of our consumption.

One of my ultimate goals is that we, as a society, live physically and emotionally liberated from our relationship with food.
To accomplish this, we must recognize our patterns, habits, associations, and relationship with food (see Chapters 12 and 13). Once we do that, we must make healthy choices to align with what our minds and bodies need for fuel versus contributing to fatigue.

Choosing nutrient-dense foods – like leafy greens, whole grains, fruits, lean meat, healthy fats, fish rich in omega-3 fatty acids, low-fat dairy products, and vegetables – give your body fuel and help heal your body.

Think about this. Since we regenerate cells every three months and nutrient-rich foods are healing, the right food choices can create a new you internally. You are changing from the inside out.

ZONING IN: THE COMFORTS OF HOME

After a long day, being home brings a sense of comfort and relief, especially if you want to escape the stress and pressures of the outside world. You may want to go numb and not think about what tomorrow will bring while watching your favorite show on television or browsing through social media.

If this is your struggle, prepare for your evenings at home by thinking ahead, which allows you to make better decisions. Choose to eat something you have a taste for, but don't overindulge.

As we learned in Chapter 12, patterns and associations crop up daily. Recognizing them is the first step to repattern. The association of going numb while doing those things with food ends up turning into therapy. **Don't allow stress relief to equal food relief.** Repattern and prepare to relax, stay connected, and make food choices that don't include calorie-laced or late-night eating.

BUT WHAT ABOUT CHOCOLATE?

Chocolate is chocolate, and there's no lighter side or healthier version of it, so try an alternative approach. Choosing a smaller portion or eating less helps. Get the small, not king-sized candy bar. Try buying a single, bite-sized portion to bring home instead of filling the candy jar with a bag of chocolate. Finally, if you're a die-hard chocolate lover, have it less frequently, on alternating nights, if your pattern/habit has been nightly.

There's a way to work everything in your life and program it in. Get creative! If you decide to eliminate your favorite snacks, you will find yourself eventually giving up and going back into your cycle.

Late-night cravings? Ask yourself, *"In 30 minutes, I'm going to bed, do I need it?"* Set a timer for 45 minutes, and if you're still awake, go ahead and eat it...if you must.

🏆 HOW TO WIN! Creating an Action Plan

The idea is not to completely overhaul your routine and schedule which can leave you feeling overwhelmed. Instead, the focus is on a plan for replacing your current routine and associations with foods that are better for your body.

Try the following:
1. Create a plan of action to trade in calorie-laced snacks for lighter and healthier options.

2. Think about what your tongue is craving and figure out how you can keep the essence of the taste or texture but have it in a way that is healthier for you.

- Are you craving salty and crunchy? Smooth and cold? Or soft and sweet?
- If you are in the mood for creamy, go for a flavored Greek yogurt instead of ice cream or do a mix of both. That means less sugar and fat, and more protein.
- If salty, crunchy is your thing, grab a handful of pretzels or air-popped popcorn. Popcorn and pretzels are less processed and at least carry some nutritional value compared to a bag of corn chips.

CHAPTER 17

THE UNHOLY TRINITY OF PRESERVATIVES: FAT, SUGAR, SODIUM

"We don't know what we don't know. Knowledge leads to having the power to make better choices."

When you're at the grocery store, look at the food label of just about any food, and chances are you'll spot a food preservative.

Preservatives are added to food to enhance their flavors, texture, or appearance, or to extend shelf life and prevent spoilage. They also can contain chemical compounds that are harmful to the body. For example, nitrates and nitrites prevent oxidation and bacterial growth, and preserve the red color in meats. However, nitrates are linked to cancer and can increase the risk of diabetes. Remember, whatever is added to any food product is added to our body when we ingest it.

Fat, sugar, and sodium are called the unholy trinity because they are the culprits contributing to chronic health conditions and weight gain as well as our food cravings. These three additives can be found in almost every product that resides on grocery store shelves. They are also present in all processed foods, in fast food, and in most frozen, canned, jarred, and boxed meals. They are everywhere!

FAT PRESERVATIVE: HYDROGENATED OIL

Hydrogenation is a process when a liquid fat is chemically changed into a solid fat by adding hydrogen. This process causes fat to be solid at room temperature. Hydrogenated oils can affect heart health because they increase "bad" (LDL) cholesterol and lower "good" (HDL) cholesterol.

Some ordinary products that are high in fat preservatives are:
- Commercially baked items
- Crackers
- Cakes
- Cookies
- Fried foods
- French fries
- Doughnuts

You can avoid hydrogenated oil by reading food labels, limiting packaged food, and choosing healthier options like baking or broiling, or opting for healthier oils like safflower, olive, or avocado. Also, avoid cooking with fats – like shortening, lard, and butter – that are solid at room temperature.

SUGAR PRESERVATIVE: HIGH FRUCTOSE CORN SYRUP

High fructose corn syrup (HFCS) is a sweetener derived from corn. The syrup is made when corn undergoes enzymatic processing in a lab to turn some of its glucose into fructose, making it sweeter. HFCS is much cheaper to process than sugar.

Additionally, the syrup's sugars are a preservative, which is why HFCS is now added to some meat.

Examples of food with high sugar preservatives are:
- Sweetened yogurt
- Salad dressing
- Cereal
- Bread

- Condiments
- Ice cream
- Syrups/jelly
- Canned vegetables
- Soups
- Lunch meats
- Pasta sauce
- Applesauce
- Soda and energy drinks

You can avoid HFCS by reading food labels, avoiding bottled, jarred, and canned products (especially condiments such as ketchup, bar-b-que sauces, and salad dressing), or packaged meals. Whenever possible, choose fresh fruits over canned.

SODIUM PRESERVATIVE: SODIUM BENZOATE

Sodium benzoate is a common type of food preservative and is the sodium salt of benzoic acid. Food manufacturers make sodium benzoate by synthesizing the compounds sodium hydroxide and benzoic acid together.

Also, sodium benzoate is found in thousands of products, even those labeled as all natural. But don't be fooled. While benzoic acid is found naturally in low levels in many fruits, the sodium benzoate listed on a product's label is synthesized in a lab.

Products containing sodium preservatives are:
- Vinegar
- Jams
- Fruit juices
- Carbonated drinks
- Canned goods
- Frozen foods/dinners

You can avoid sodium benzoate by reading food labels, decreasing the amount of processed food you eat, and choosing food with natural ingredients.

🏆 HOW TO WIN! Eating Foods Without Preservatives

If it feels like the contents of your pantry and cupboard could use a makeover, try the following to cut down (and eliminate) the preservatives you are eating:

- Read product labels carefully. Keep an eye out for strange-sounding ingredients.
- Change your family's weekly menus to focus on freshly prepared meals made with simple, wholesome ingredients.
- Peruse old-fashioned cookbooks for interesting recipes. If your favorite recipes call for canned soups, saltine crackers, or other processed ingredients, alter the recipes to include healthier ingredients.
- Shop for fresh, whole foods at farmers' markets or organic grocery stores. Organic foods rarely have preservatives. Locally grown produce needs to be shipped only short distances to reach consumers, making preservatives unnecessary.
- Buy fresh cuts of meat instead of cured meats or lunch meat, which contain a lot of salt as a preservative. Make sure the cuts are lean to reduce the amount of saturated fat in your diet.
- Introduce more whole grains like bulgur wheat, barley, and brown rice to your family's diet. Add freshly cooked legumes like chickpeas, kidney beans, and pinto beans.
- Season foods with dried herbs and flavorful spices rather than packaged mixes, which typically contain salt, artificial flavoring, and added preservatives.

CHAPTER 18

EAT LIKE YOUR METABOLISM

"Skipping meals is like stealing gas from your tank. Your metabolism slows down, and fewer calories are burned. Eat small meals frequently to fuel the furnace, increase your metabolism, and burn more calories."

Metabolism is the process by which our bodies convert what we eat into the energy we need to survive.

Did you know your metabolism is highest during the day and lowest at night?

Picture a tornado that is wide at the top and narrow toward the bottom. That's the shape of your metabolism. First thing in the morning, it's moving quickly around the highest point at the top of the funnel. Then, as the day progresses, your metabolism moves down the funnel, slowing as it heads to the narrow end at the bottom.

Knowing that your metabolism is highest during the day and lower at night means you can plan your meals and food intake to better align with how quickly or slowly your body will burn it off. Try having more calorie-heavy meals when your metabolism is moving faster so you can burn off the calories.

This is what we mean by "eat like your metabolism."

You may have been taught that to lose weight, you must eat fewer calories. But the opposite is true. If you consume fewer calories, your body's metabolism will naturally slow down because it thinks it is starving. It goes into conservation mode for survival. When this happens, you might not feel hungry throughout the day.

Remember, you want to feel hunger pangs. Hunger means that your metabolism is kicking into gear, and your body's running low on energy. When you feel hungry, you can answer your body by giving it the fuel it's asking for.

THE EVENING DILEMMA
The evening can be the most critical point of your day. This is the time where you are finally home, you are decompressing after a long day, and getting ready to relax in front of the TV.

If you're like many others, evenings are a time when your defenses are at the lowest and when you are more susceptible to react to the day's stress. So, guess what! You reach for the snacks! Remember that during the evening, your metabolism is nearing its slowest point, and your body will not have the ability to burn any extra calories.

EVERY BODY'S DIFFERENT
It is important to remember everyone is different, and metabolisms will vary from person to person. Gender, age, level of physical activity, state of health, and genetics play a role in your metabolic rate. Don't compare yourself to the next person. Focus on what your body needs. The goal is to get your body on a cycle in which it is expecting food more frequently. And once it does, your body will let you know when it is ready to eat! Just make sure you are feeding it the right fuel!

BOB'S STORY

Many clients have begun to understand how to adjust their eating patterns during the right time of the day. My favorite story is about Bob. Bob used to eat once a day and would drink coffee from morning to lunch. Also, he ate late at night and went right to bed after his meal. He was mystified about why he couldn't lose weight.

I talked to him about his eating habits and told him that eating one meal a day doesn't provide enough fuel for his body and slows his metabolism. His eating habits caused his body to switch into conservation mode to survive with little to no fueling. Furthermore, his body could not use those late-night calories efficiently and converted them to fat.

We worked on solutions and changed his eating patterns. We also incorporated more food than he was initially comfortable with. He started with a balanced breakfast and added light snacks in between lunch and a small dinner.

Now that he has been eating throughout the day, he doesn't feel ravenous at night. Within a few weeks, he was amazed at how hungry he was throughout the day and how quickly his body adapted to the change.

He was also surprised at his initial 10-pound weight loss and how his energy level had increased. I reminded him that his new eating habits gave his body the fuel it needed at the right time. His increased metabolism was a by-product of this action.

He became a believer and went on to lose 30 more pounds over the next few months.

🏆 HOW TO WIN! Creating a Metabolic Eating Plan

- Let your food mimic your metabolism by eating higher-calorie foods earlier in the day.
- Don't skip breakfast because it can jumpstart your metabolism for the day.
- Don't overeat at night when your metabolism is slower.
- If you decide to eat the sugary snack or savory treat, opt to have it earlier when your body can metabolize it quicker.
- Remember at night and when you are asleep, your metabolism is at its lowest. Therefore, your body cannot burn those calories as efficiently as it does during the day when you are awake.
- Physical activity is like giving yourself metabolism boosters. The more you exercise, the more you help your body burn calories.

CHAPTER 19

FACING TEMPTATIONS: SECOND (AND THIRD) HELPINGS

"When you are facing a tasty temptation and want to go for that second serving, think: Eat what my body needs, not just what I want."

Stopping yourself from digging into seconds (or even thirds) isn't always easy. Then when you overdo it, you beat yourself up with feelings of guilt and negative self-talk.

OWNING THAT YOU WANT MORE
You will always want more so telling yourself you don't is falsifying how you feel. Own the fact that you want more. Then ask yourself, *"Am I hungry?" "Is this second helping what my body needs or simply what I want?"* Asking these questions will put you back on track.

If you're like most people, you may not listen to your body's hunger signals. When your body is hungry, your stomach will growl, you won't feel energetic, or you may have difficulty concentrating. If you don't have physical symptoms of hunger, you may be bored or stressed.

Always remember, everything is a mindset. When confronted with second helpings and you aren't hungry, think through your choices and remind yourself of your purpose and focus on the bigger picture. Overeating will only contribute to short-lived satisfaction, unnecessary calories, and unwanted weight.

💬 LAURA'S STORY

Laura's a client who I am fond of just as much as she is fond of carrot cake. Throughout her life, carrot cake with icing has been her weakness. She told me a story of when she attended her cousin's wedding and found herself having three slices of carrot cake.

I asked her why she found it challenging to have only one slice.

She hesitated and then shared how she felt the need to keep eating it because she wanted to keep the taste in her mouth. She talked about how much she loved everything about the cake: the texture, the smell, the taste.

I told her that when we overindulge, we satisfy one 1x2 muscle, our tongue. It's five minutes of pleasure, and the rest of your body (and mind) takes the brunt of it. We go backward from our healthier eating goals, both emotionally and physically.

You must ask yourself if it's worth it.

Laura realized that she was temporarily satisfied, but the emotional and physical discontent lasted ten times longer. On her next encounter with carrot cake, she decided that her body deserved better and having one slice was enough to satisfy her tongue.

🏆 HOW TO WIN! Passing on Seconds (or Thirds)

If your body doesn't need it, choose to leave it. Consider the following strategies for winning the fight against temptation.
- Ask yourself, *"Does my body deserve to live in an environment where overeating is the norm?"*
- Tell yourself that the second or third serving will place you in a position of feeling defeated and out of control. It won't solve any problems and will create more challenges.
- Remind yourself that balance means one and done, not two and a few.
- See yourself as a work in progress. If you find that second helpings disappeared from your plate, don't beat yourself up. Whatever brought you to that extra piece will happen again if you don't remember to ask, tell, and remind yourself.
- Love yourself and your body. Even though three helpings might sound incredible, having three servings will affect how you feel about yourself and will set you back from the goals you want to reach.

CHAPTER 20
FINAL NUTS AND BOLTS

"Don't let susceptibilities be your downfall."

Now that you know a little more about the importance of water, using food for fuel, eating for your metabolism, and avoiding temptation, it's time to make a plan for eating and know that some days will be easier than others.

KNOW YOUR SCHEDULE – PLAN TO EAT!
Hectic days and idle days are both challenging, even though they are on opposite sides of the spectrum.

On chaotic days, it's easy to get caught up and forget to eat. Since you know what's in store, plan ahead by having a quick shake, keeping simple snacks close by, and creating a go-to plan for lunch. For example: Packing a lunch is a great option, placing a pre-order for a salad to be delivered, or scouting out a close restaurant that serves healthy food, and setting your alarm to go there at a specified time, will be beneficial to your day and overall goals.

On idle days, it's easy to go with the flow and graze all day. Plan ahead and surround yourself with low-calorie snacks, veggies, and food that won't pack high numbers of calories each time you grab for it.

Every day you will eat. Don't wing it. You are your priority. Scheduling your food according to your days is one of the surest ways to keep synchronized and successful despite stress, changes, or extremes.

You know your habits, and you know what you are susceptible to. Plan your days.

PASS OR FAIL MENTALITY – DON'T SUCCUMB TO IT!
Don't judge yourself by pass-fail or all-in or all-out. Part of the human experience is making mistakes. Part of being mature and successful is learning from mistakes and doing something different as a result.

On your next road trip instead of defaulting to stopping at the nearest fast-food restaurant or gas station, pack your snacks so you are prepared.

At the next office party, choose to place less food on your plate than the last time. During the next birthday party, eat less this year. For the upcoming holiday season, eat small healthy meals before you go so you aren't tempted to eat foods that don't align with your goals, and so you aren't subjected to what is being served because you're hungry.

Hiccups happen when you are working on your plan. This doesn't mean you've failed. Keep focused on your strategy. Being intentional will keep you encouraged to meet your desired outcomes through challenges.

It's not about passing or failing. It's about growing. Did you know:
- The lowest sugar fruits are all berries (for example, strawberries, blueberries, raspberries, and blackberries). The highest sugar fruits are dried fruit, bananas, grapes, and figs.
- Chewing gum is the best alternative after a meal, if you have a sweet tooth, or if you are bored. It changes your taste buds and keeps you busy.

- The only thing "sugar-free" and "fat-free" is water!
- "Fat-free" usually means added sugar. "Sugar-free" usually means added artificial sugar. Instead, look for labels that say low fat or low sugar, and choose these options.

FINAL THOUGHTS

We all have areas in our lives that we'd like to improve. When it comes to food, the goal is to recognize challenges or downfalls and then create a game plan. For example, if your downfall is not enough time, create a "plan ahead" solution. If your downfall is being bored, figure out the remedy to prevent idle eating. Then, refrain from labeling weak areas as problems and start seeking solutions. **Vulnerable areas will remain as such if you never address them.**

Finally, remember that healthy eating is not a black or white, pass or fail experience. Create some grey space. Look at your wins and be determined to face your soft spots, so you have solid ground to stand on.

PART V
Six Game Plans That Really Work

Overcoming Challenges

Making Progress

Repositioning Yourself

Seeing Food as a Tool

Knowing the Difference

Giving Yourself Validation

"I ain't Martin Luther King. I don't need a dream. I have a plan."

Spike Lee

CHAPTER 21

#1 CHALLENGES ARE INEVITABLE – YOU'LL PREVAIL

"The moment you begin to compromise your time or efforts, is the moment you must snap back and say, 'No, I am my priority.' Always remind yourself of your needs."

It would be a lie and say you won't face times of sadness, frustration, and distraction. These challenges are a part of living. You will experience times where you don't feel your best, or you feel stagnant. There will be times when eating another salad is the last thing you want to do. There will also be times when you've had one too many drinks, and your inhibitions went out the window.

But this does not mean you aren't strong enough to keep going. This only means you are going through a temporary phase, challenging though it may be.

Recognize when you are in a challenging situation. **Refuse to give up on yourself and push through relentlessly.** It's likely a short-term situation.

You will not always be motivated. When that happens, remember your goals, focus on what's in your best interest, keep your feet planted, and remember the solid foundation you've built.

Appreciating your victories and acknowledging the challenges will help you to get back on track and prevail.

FOOD IS OUR CONSTANT – INTAKE SHOULDN'T BE DICTATED BY CIRCUMSTANCES

Food is there during the highest and lowest times of our lives. Food is there when you're celebrating a promotion, graduation, birth, or wedding. Food is there when you've gotten fired, lost a family member, broken up, or are going through a divorce. The danger is that when we experience these highs and lows, we go to extremes with our food choices/amounts as well. It's accepted in society that most will gain weight during the holidays and eat a pint (or two) of ice cream when life gets stressful.

So many times we set ourselves up at the cost of "one-day defeats," which have turned into weeks of indulgences, resulting in five to 15-pound packages around our hips, thighs, and stomachs. We have to stop letting external circumstances control our lives.

"There will be struggles along the way but keeping self-care in the forefront will allow you to prevail in the end; after all, you are worth it."

CHAPTER 22

#2 PRACTICE MEANS PROGRESS

"Changing what you've always done takes being focused on progress, not perfection."

When deciding to make changes, we would like the transition to be flawless, with the idea that to become successful, it's necessary to be perfect. There is immense pressure to get everything "right" the first time, so if you make a mistake, it's tempting to give up because perfection is the expectation.

Planning to be perfect is setting yourself up to fail because perfection is subjective. Because everyone has different ideas of what perfect means, we find ourselves on an endless quest of judgment and failed expectations. Replace judgment and failed expectations with "grace."

Then, practice grace with discipline.

GRACE WITH DISCIPLINE
Grace is understanding that you will make mistakes and that your mistakes don't define you. Knowing that mistakes are inevitable, take the pressure off yourself, acknowledging that mistakes are simply part of the process. Then use what happened to make new choices as you shift your view of yourself and as you reach your goals.

Progress is the alternative to perfection. **Practice means progress.** When you take on new tasks, it will take making and overcoming mistakes, time, patience, and grace to progress and be successful. As you are graciously allowing yourself to be human, you are also implementing discipline in your actions.

Discipline guides you and helps you focus as you move toward your goals. The application of discipline is not to create such high standards that you feel overwhelmed. Discipline means keeping steady during the process of accomplishment.

And discipline is relative. For example, if you usually grab three cookies after dinner, an applied discipline can be choosing two cookies instead. That's a win!

If you have decided to begin walking every week, discipline means deciding to walk two or four times a week. Whichever you choose, as long as you walk, and stick to your choice, you are progressing and exhibiting discipline.

"Practice means progress. Give yourself grace and maintain the practice of discipline."

CHAPTER 23
#3 REPOSITION YOURSELF

> *"If in the past you've felt controlled by certain foods, it's time to change that."*

Repositioning means changing your mindset from victim to decision-maker. Too often we've given our power to food instead of using our power to decide which foods we will consume.

Have you felt powerless, saying to yourself or anyone who would listen, *"It's calling my name." "I can't say no!" "I'll try just a couple." "It's my favorite."* Or *"I get weak, I can't help it!"*

All these statements mean you have been placing something with no authority over your choices, rendering you powerless. It's time to reclaim your power.

Reclaiming your power means changing your perspective and your self-talk. Changing your words to, *"I'm making this decision." "I'm choosing which foods to eat; they are not choosing me." "I am strong enough to say yes and powerful enough to say no."*

Once these statements become part of your new language, your position shifts to the offense. And that's where you want to be.

> *"You are responsible for what you think, say, and for what you choose to eat. Your thoughts and words give you the power to stand in a position of authority. Reposition yourself and claim your power."*

CHAPTER 24

#4 SEE FOOD NOT AS A TOOL BUT AS NUTRITION

"Choosing a better relationship with food and exercise means having a better relationship with yourself and with your health."

How many times have you lost weight and found it again three months later?

If your definition of success is changing what you see in the mirror, you will find yourself in a perpetual state of being unfulfilled. Stop making every decision in the name of weight, looks, acceptance, compliments, and approval. Stop focusing on calories or eliminating certain foods in the name of vanity just to fit in – to fit into that dress, that crowd, or for those vacations. Grueling workouts, yoyo diets, deprivation, and calorie counting alone usually mean short-lived changes to the physical body. This practice means you are using food and exercise as tools instead of nutrition and wellness.

Attaining your body goals takes far more than focusing on the outside; it takes seeing food and yourself differently and recognizing what's most important. Remember, practicing self-love and self-care means being reflective, proactive, and making consistent changes to support your overall vitality.

Yes, your food and exercise are ways to modify your body, but they are more than just tools. Your nutrition and exercise should be a representation of who you are, not only devices to make a change. The acts of eating nutrients and exercising are affirming your desire to provide your body the opportunity to be at its best.

Begin to view strawberries and fish as nutrients. Choose to move your body because doing so keeps you strong and vital. Focus on making changes to your nutrition and movement as an extension of who you are instead of tools needed to get the job done.

"Internal change creates external results."

CHAPTER 25

#5 KNOW THE DIFFERENCE: FOOD VS. NUTRITION

"Food is your mood. Nutrition is your intention"

Food, by definition, is any substance that we eat or drink to maintain life and growth.

Nutrition is the act or process of obtaining the food necessary for health and growth. Allow yourself to see food differently and associate it with nutrients. If your usual food choices aren't particularly nutritious, reconsider what you eat.

Think about the first time you met your meant-to-be best friend. Before you knew them, they were a person living a life, but they were utterly unknown to you. Once you met them, you engaged with them and built a rapport. Also, you must've had some mutual respect for you to now identify as "best friends." As a matter of fact, best friends are reflections of who you are – how you see yourself, everyday activities and interests, what you value, and what you aspire to be.

Let's take the same approach to our foods.

When you label food as nutrients, it's like giving a person a name. Now this "food" has meaning and significance. You have defined it for its value, such as you do your best friend. For example, when you decide to make a trip to your favorite hamburger and fries place, I am sure you don't say, *"Let's go to the Greasiest Spoon to order some nutrients."* But essentially, that's what you're doing. You are putting the by-products of the greasy spoons into your body when you eat from that place. When you think of it this way, it's easier to change your associations.

By changing your language, you can quickly discern the difference between what are nutrients and what are not.

I have spent most of my adulthood and profession learning and understanding how nutrition contributes to all aspects of our lives. In my view, nutrition is life. Without it, we would not be here. As you grow and educate yourself about nutrition, you will find a new respect for what you eat. Let your words define the way you see your choices and let your choices determine the way you see yourself.

"Say no to greasy spoons and yes to nutrients."

CHAPTER 26

#6 GIVE YOURSELF VALIDATION

"Don't allow the scale to determine or undermine your value."

In the past, you have been trained to find validation in weight loss. Watching the scale dictates our mood and self-esteem. The scale is not neutral, therefore running back to it is not the way to live. Don't live off the scale.

The source of validation should come from how you treat yourself, stemming from your relationship with yourself. Every time you make a healthy choice, you are validating yourself. When you focus on taking care of yourself, the by-product of physical change follows, the unnecessary weight falls off, and your body heals itself from the inside out. That is the way to live.

"Nutrition is self-care. Nutrition is self-love. Nutrition is you."

PART VI
What It Takes to Win

Finding Motivation

Pursuing Consistency

"The more time you spend contemplating what you should have done...you lose valuable time planning what you can and will do."

Lil Wayne

CHAPTER 27

MOTIVATION IS A GOOD STARTER, BUT ...

There are days when you won't feel motivated, but you have to do 'it' anyway.

Have you ever been motivated by an inspirational song or a persuasive speech? Have you ever depended on motivation to get started or to keep going? The interesting thing about motivation is that it isn't constant. Motivation is meant to light a fire, not to keep a blaze burning. Motivation comes in spurts.

WHAT HAPPENS WHEN MOTIVATION ISN'T THERE?
Society has trained us to believe that motivation is needed to move forward, but we are not taught how to live, or how to make progress when we are not motivated. So, when you proclaim that you must be motivated, you are already setting yourself up for failure.

You will not always be motivated to get to the gym or to prepare a healthy meal. When you're not motivated, you can comfortably kick your workout or your healthier food choices to next week and fall back into old habits.

The trick is to recognize that you're not motivated and separating motivation from your choice. Instead, remember your goals and be committed to them. Also, take the steps to complete the tasks to reach your objectives.

That separation from (not) being motivated and making a choice to be successful by accomplishing those tasks means you are making progress, significant progress.

I think about it like doing laundry or yard work. I am not motivated to do any of it, but it needs to be done. So, once I acknowledge that I'm not motivated, I change my mindset and do the work anyway.

💬 SANDY'S STORY

A few years ago, my client, Sandy, said, *"I need an event or vacation to be motivated to change."* She felt that if she had a deadline to hit, she would be motivated and have something to work toward.

There are a few ways to look at this. First, Sandy only felt the need to be healthy or to lose weight because she wanted to have a healthy "look" for temporary reasons. So, it was expected that right after she met her goal, she was either going to return to old habits or try to find new motivation. Second, Sandy felt motivation was the only way she could act. She continued to live in a cycle of weight gain and weight loss. She hadn't figured out that motivation was her downfall.

Maybe this is a common challenge that you have faced in your life.

To address Sandy's challenges, we took a step back to understand what motivation means and how it works. I explained that motivation is like a fire that goes out unless it's rekindled.

Sandy needed something steady and enduring instead of the ebb and flow of motivation. I explained that she could operate without being motivated. To do this, she had to let everything go and get used to making the best choice when it was the last thing she wanted to do.

At the time, Sandy was in law school. I asked her about how motivated she was to write papers, prepare for the next class lecture, and study long nights. She admitted that she was not motivated to do any of it but knew it needed to be done. She had to shift her mindset to make it happen. And every night for three years, that's the mindset she had.

I pointed out that this was the perfect example to show herself that she had the capability of getting things done without motivation. She just never made it a part of her eating choices.

She realized that depending on motivation would never get her where she wants to be, and perhaps it was an excuse not to put healthier choices into practice.

Over time, she began to change her perspective, language, and actions. Of course, it wasn't easy, but she recognized that being motivated was short-lived, and she wanted more for herself.

We worked through these obstacles one at a time, and she now can make choices that benefit her best, and not because her next vacation is just around the corner.

🏆 HOW TO WIN! Finding Your Motivation

On this journey, plan well, set your intentions, and remember to take it day by day. Circumstances will change, and so will your situations and levels of motivation. Look at what's driving you, especially in those moments when you don't "feel like" taking that extra step or completing that task. Because motivation comes in spurts, don't rely on it to start or achieve your goals.

When you can't find your motivation, try these strategies:
- Remember your *Why* and the purpose behind what you're trying to accomplish.
- Create a plan that is realistic and feels rewarding. Break your goal(s) into smaller, manageable steps.
- Keep a positive mental attitude. Positive thoughts lead to positive actions.
- View tasks as an opportunity to take a different approach. Tackle procrastination by not making excuses. Talk yourself right back into doing what's best for you!
- Remove distractions and temptations.
- Choose success by creating a mental picture of yourself completing a task. Then, stick to your choices and see them manifest and feel success.
- Acknowledge your wins after completing tasks or reaching milestones.
- Tell yourself that with every positive choice you make you are succeeding.
- Keep talking to yourself and keep flourishing!

CHAPTER 28
PURSUE CONSISTENCY

"Motivation is a good starter, but it's not what's going to keep you consistent. Commit to doing 'it' no matter what. Say no to motivation and yes to consistency."

Motivation can stimulate action and is often strong when you're excited but quickly wears off when things get hard. On the other hand, consistency is slow-paced and long-lasting, allowing you to achieve results over time.

CONSISTENCY LEADS TO HABITS AND ACTIONS
I get it, consistency can be difficult to practice, but we do it every day, often without realizing it. We get up in the morning to go to work. We have dinner at a set time. We walk the dog in the afternoon. We have routines that we follow every day. Consistency leads to habits, and habits form actions.

But consistency can work for you or against you. For example, if you consistently eat three doughnuts every morning with your two cups of coffee containing six packets of sugar, you will begin to look like the doughnut in terms of roundness and fluffiness. Do you like those results? To reach your goals, you must practice consistency to successfully create a solid foundation for anything worthy or valuable in life.

Consistency is the achievement of a level of performance that maintains its quality over time. In other words, the quality is the same because you are doing things the same way, having the same standard over time.

CONSISTENCY BECOMES EASIER OVER TIME

I am sure you have said starting a new endeavor is easy, but keeping it going is the hard part. Here is the beauty of consistency; it builds over time and becomes easier if you allow yourself to stick to it.

What does it take to get to the other side of a brick wall? Consider your process. If you use your will power, energy, and force to bulldoze through a brick wall, you may get through to the other side, but then you're worn out, depleted, exhausted, burnt out, and over-exerted. But you've made it to the other side.

If you had the same wall and I said, *"Here is a small pick. I want you to chisel your way through the wall."* Looking at the wall and holding the chisel, you know this will take a very long time, but you decide to go for it. You chisel and chisel making small gains, but this act of constant chiseling becomes routine over time.

Dieting is much like bulldozing. Taking a drastic route to reach a goal, pushing your way through and meeting the goal, you feel as if your mission is accomplished and you are finally done! The wall is down, the weight is gone, and you stop working because you broke through. Right? You're proud, but you're exhausted, and when you're tired, it's easy to retreat, falling back into old habits and patterns. That's why bulldozing and dieting don't work over the long term.

Instead, think about weight loss and healthier living choices through chiseling rather than trying to force changes. When you chisel, you are practicing consistency through small gains. Eventually, the practice of consistency becomes natural, and you find yourself progressing without realizing it has turned into your everyday thing. The wall that you are working to break down will eventually crumble, and your constant chiseling will continue because you have turned it into a habit. And you will not be exhausted and feel it's time to stop because you've met your goals. **When you practice consistency, you can find strength and endurance in the process.**

💬 CASSIE'S STORY

When Cassie and I first met, she had a goal to lose 65 pounds. And the only way she knew how to lose the weight and feel successful was to jump on the latest quick-fix program. Anxious to shed the pounds, she had given herself six months to reach her goal. The result was that she fixated on doing whatever it took to force the weight off. If that meant fasting, removing every carb from every meal, or drinking only meal replacements, she did it.

After meeting over a few months, Cassie realized that her biggest struggle was learning how to be consistent. She said, *"I don't have a problem starting, but it's hard to keep going."*

I asked her why she felt that consistency was a struggle for her.

She shared that she didn't know how to maintain consistency once she started a new program for change. Furthermore, she was taught an "all or none" philosophy. If she wasn't 100% successful, she failed.

I quickly debunked that statement, telling her that the all-or-none mentality is a self-defeating way to handle any change. There will be ups and downs as one learns new patterns and transitions to a new way of living.

To help Cassie, we worked together on strategies for being consistent. We started with small steps like exchanging fruit for chips and water for juice. It took six weeks for her to feel consistent. Next, Cassie worked on reducing soda intake and adding veggies to every dinner meal.

Through this process, she learned that the act of consistency is essential, not what she is consistent at.

By getting used to being consistent and building her confidence, Cassie slowly (very slowly) incorporated more changes. And she began losing weight quickly because she wasn't forcing the process and was off the start-stop cycle. Over time, she found it easier to grab a piece of fruit and bottled water instead of a bag of chips and soda. Now, she has veggies with every meal.

Cassie continues to chisel and break down her walls one choice at a time. And she doesn't feel overwhelmed and exhausted. She discovered that her weight-loss success wouldn't happen by force. Instead, it will occur with patience and consistency.

🏆 HOW TO WIN! Creating Consistent Action

Consistency – and consistent action – is a vital ingredient for achieving success. If you find yourself running out of steam, follow the steps below to keep moving forward.
1. Be clear about your intention.
2. Don't bulldoze, but chisel your way through.
3. Consider your process. Change takes time, so embrace the time it takes.
4. Set achievable goals and make a single change that can multiply into more.
5. Use motivation only as a starter, then shift to consistency.
6. When you feel unmotivated, choose to do "it" anyway.
7. Keep striving. Remember that you are stronger than you think.
8. Practice is like taking steady steps to reach your goals. And the process will get easier when you are consistent.

PART VII
Inspiration for Fighting Your Best Fight

Envisioning Liberation

Taking Your Best Shot

Learning to Fish

Believing in Yourself

"The reason most people never reach their goals is that they don't define them, or ever seriously consider them as believable or achievable. Winners can tell you where they are going, what they plan to do along the way, and who will be sharing the adventure with them."

Denis Waitley

CHAPTER 29

MY HOPE FOR YOU IS LIBERATION

"Be aware of your environment, and its impact on your choices."

When I was in college, I was known as "the hair girl." I was that person on campus who braided, twisted, and styled hair. As most people know, excellent stylists are also typically good listeners, confidantes, and serve as therapists for their clients.

After putting the finishing touches on the perfect styles, I watched as my clients would step into the restroom with their makeup, apply it, and walk out like a whole new person. They had a new awareness, a pep in their step, and genuinely felt good about themselves as a result of having their crowns beautifully coifed. Knowing I contributed to that sense of wellbeing gave me a sense of pride and purpose, which made me want to make more significant contributions.

So, I became a dietitian. After passing my exams, I was qualified to help people make changes beyond the surface of their hair and more in-depth than their outward appearance. My goal is to provide guidance to self-awareness, self-actualization, and – ultimately – liberation.

Once you leave life-long struggles, pain, and counterproductive habits to your health behind, you never have to be captive to your past. I know how it feels to love myself and consistently show self-love by treating my body well.

That's what I want you to know and feel – liberation. Liberation is freedom. Liberation is that feeling of not limiting yourself. It's the precursor to embodying the courage to live into the life you deserve and want for yourself.

My definition of liberation and happiness will be different from yours. However, it is a universal feeling I am sure we would all like to relate to, even if we haven't yet.

Think about this. Have you ever removed the doors of a Jeep and experienced the joy of riding in an open vehicle?

Picture yourself driving a jeep with your arm extended and leg hanging out the open door. Imagine the freedom to jump in and out of the vehicle without the extra step of opening a door. And the freedom to breathe fresh air! The Jeep also can go onto rocky terrain where most cars aren't equipped to travel. Visualize having the freedom to roam on unpaved roads, loose dirt, unleveled pathways, and over rolling hills that would be obstacles under other circumstances.

You experience the greatest joy because you're equipped and brave enough to experience all that the vehicle offers, while trusting yourself over every twist and turn. Along with this, you have enough structure (discipline and desire), to keep the Jeep – and yourself – on the road and in safe territory as you continue to move forward on your journey.

Liberation feels like this! You *can* be free to live a life that is unencumbered. You deserve that.

Once you've experienced liberation, you will want everyone else to live freely as well. Living in freedom comes with a feeling of content that overrides external influences. Liberation is not superficial or insignificant. You no longer depend on the number on the scale to determine your worth. You no longer struggle to resist a spread of desserts or week-long holiday feasts. You will see food as nutrition, and your relationship will remain profoundly rooted and intact. You feel your best without pangs of guilt.

WITH LIBERATION COMES CLARITY OF PURPOSE

As you are envisioning the way liberation looks and feels, consider the struggles it took to get there. I will not lie. It's going to be a rocky road, and I don't mean ice cream!

The path may be long and lonely. It will test what you genuinely want for yourself. You will be tempted to stop or stall. However, I encourage you to get started. Don't wait until later. Then, appreciate every step you take on your journey. Embrace your efforts. As you move forward, you are building the strength that comes from endurance. **And your endurance increases every day with every choice you make in alignment with your goals.**

CHAPTER 30
YOU'VE GOT ONE SHOT!

"You've got one life to live. Shoot your best shot today and every day! That's how you will get the life you want to live. You must prove you are stronger than the voice telling you it's not worth it or you can't do it. Make a solid plan, follow through, and put yourself first."

Ask yourself, *"If I have one chance to make the best choice for my health and happiness, why do I flounder?"*

If you are like many others, floundering is the result of our choices not aligned with our health goals. We, often unintentionally, abuse our bodies by filling them with harmful food. We sigh or whine the moment someone suggests a healthy meal. We procrastinate about moving our bodies the way they are meant to move. Ultimately, we routinely gamble with our lives and health, deciding to look the other way and ignoring that our poor choices lower our quality of life.

When meeting with clients either individually or in group sessions, I ask them how long they have struggled with their weight and self-image. Most say their entire life. When I ask, *"What would it feel like if you overcame the obstacles that have been plaguing you?"* There's usually a long, awkward pause. Most people don't know how to respond because they haven't envisioned that as a possibility.

Can you imagine waking up in the morning thinking, feeling, and knowing that, *"This is the day I must shoot my shot because I won't get another chance"?*

If you lived like you had one shot at living your best life, you'd likely live more boldly, courageously, and urgently. You get one life, and you don't get a second chance to experience it. What matters is what you do with the time you are given. Life doesn't provide a sequel to re-live it a different way. You can choose to do and live differently.

Wouldn't it be remarkable if you not only overcame this lifelong struggle, but you also realized how strong and mighty you are? Perhaps you would take this newfound strength and apply it to areas of your life? Being liberated gives confidence and the audacity to go for that promotion you know you deserve, leave a relationship that was holding you back, or to become a more patient parent who helps their child recognize their fullest potential.

Do you see how this is connected? As you become better and more confident, you can then spread it outward to other areas of your life. You have been through the hard work and self-realization and now you believe in yourself.

CHAPTER 31

ONCE YOU'VE LEARNED TO FISH – KEEP FISHING

"Having the tools to change is one thing but being confident and determined to use them is another."

Success is a constant pursuit. The idea of success doesn't mean your work is done now that you've finally shed the excess weight, or your glucose levels are back within normal ranges. That would be temporary; a short-lived celebration. I hope that in three to four years, you will have continued your work, optimized your health, maintained your weight, and are living confidently because of your consistent choices.

SEE YOURSELF FOR WHO YOU WANT TO BE
Every day you have a choice to become who you truly are, or you can settle for what you have been in the past. You are equipped with the tools and knowledge to create what you desire successfully. Often success in one area leads to success in other regions because achievements will fuel your fire to want more. Remember to measure your success and track your progress!

To live up to your potential and promise, explore and experience new things. I've known adults who have returned to school to finish or begin degrees. Others have been able to reconnect with relatives because they've let go of past hurts and judgments, while others have enjoyed running so much that they've become serial marathoners!

It's time to become the person you want to be. Success is right around the corner, and I know you possess the courage to make the necessary changes to accomplish your goals!

KEEP YOUR MINDSET SHARP

When you know who you want to be, you must keep your mindset sharp and aligned with your goals.

Think about when you use a knife. You need to keep its edges sharp to prevent it from getting dull and less effective. When you sharpen a knife, it doesn't change the shape but allows it to function at full capacity.

Apply the same concept to your new routine. To maintain success, you must check to make sure that your new mindset remains focused and sharp, so you don't revert to negative self-talk, procrastination, feelings of failure, or disappointment.

Also, a sharp mindset will help you to be proactive during the tough, stressful, and unpredictable times. If situations don't go as planned, that doesn't mean things are falling apart. Instead, you may have to refocus. Think of it as an opportunity to reflect on the impact of your decisions and how to make better choices.

BE CONFIDENT IN YOUR CHOICES

As you begin to manifest your relationship with food, it will be evident. You will look, walk, and act differently. Also, your energy will be felt by those around you. People may see the pep in your step and want some of what you have because they sense your newfound freedom. When you unapologetically choose the smoked fish with steamed veggies on the side instead of a burger or steak platter, they will notice.

Which leads me to say, *"Stand up for your food choices!"* There's no reason to justify your decisions with anyone. Standing up for what you want doesn't mean explaining or boasting. Standing up means being confident in your choices. Your foods and your preferences represent who you are. **Standing up for your food means standing up for yourself.** Instead of making comments, people will ask what you've been doing to shine from within. Stand up, be a leader in your choices, and you will find that others will follow.

Your decision to make good nutrition a part of your life can be a vehicle to success in other areas. The strategies you learn to transform your mindset can be applied to other challenges that require focus and patience.

> ### 💬 KARLA'S STORY
>
> Karla is a mother of two girls, one diagnosed with autism. Even though she's happily married with a successful career, Karla has struggled to take care of her family, hold a managerial position at work, and find balance for herself. When we met, her weight gain reflected her struggles.
>
> We worked together to fine-tune her nutrition decisions, worked through obstacles standing in the way of success, and focused on finding her time.
>
> Eventually, she lost 20 pounds and changed her body composition dramatically. This process took 10 to 12 months, but every time we met, she had made further steps forward. She worked through obstacles and invested in her personal life.
>
> Over time and after many resets, Karla began to have a clearer vision. She developed tools to be proactive, better understand nutrition, and establish rooted *Why* reasons. When our time together ended, she had more energy, was able to focus at work, and had control of life's challenges.

Eventually, her entire family began eating healthier, and Karla saw positive improvements in her daughters. By feeding them more natural foods, their behaviors and learning ability improved. Karla also moved with more confidence and was ready to face unexpected circumstances that would have sent her into a spiral six months ago. She added more exercise to her routine and accepted a job promotion. Additionally, she has the energy to play with her daughters now. Karla is a prime example of how one can apply lessons and tools learned for change to other areas of life.

She feels good in her clothes and will never go on another diet because her lifestyle has changed. Now, Karla is experiencing the success of hard work. She's living in liberation and is never going back!

THE POWER OF YOUR INFLUENCE

Once you have had a taste of success, you might want those around you to experience it too. Proof that you are living in your success happens when you start hearing people say the words you remember saying. *"I have to get back on my diet,"* *"This is my birthday, so I am going to do what I want,"* or *"I will get back on board when my kids start back into their school year."*

Only this time, you will listen with compassion, not judgment, because you were once there.

You influence by your actions and by telling your story. It takes being personable by relating and discussing ways that worked for you. Your patience and support will allow others to choose to change for themselves when they are ready. Many times, people seem apprehensive about change; however, they might not understand what the journey looks like.

You can be an advocate for transformation.

First, listen to what they are going through to support them as they are making changes. Then, nudge and find subtle ways to challenge them to get their wheels turning. You might ask them, *"What makes you feel so vulnerable around certain foods?" "When was the last time you used your gym membership or went out for a routine walk?"* These provoking questions can make people think. Then, you can work together to find a solution.

Don't be offended if the person replies defensively or makes excuses when asked questions. The best way to be helpful is to create suggestions. Discuss how you found it hard to readjust your schedule or how you were able to find two mornings during the week to take early morning exercise classes. Your suggestions might spark ideas.

Think about where you were when you started and where you are today. How many times did it take you to begin your journey? Who influenced you, and how did you feel? Did you feel judged or forced? Or did you feel supported?

When talking to someone who is just starting the process of change, you may have to take a slow, subtle approach.

HELPING OTHERS LEARN TO FISH

When you help others learn to fish, you are giving them the tools for creating lasting change. You lead by example as well as through the conversations you have.

Consider a scenario where you are out to dinner with a friend, colleague, or significant other. Typically, at the end of the meal, you each ordered dessert. Instead of ordering separate plates of a high-calorie delicacy, you suggest a dessert you can share. Or you may recommend visiting a nearby coffee shop to enjoy a cup of coffee and skip dessert altogether.

- You have taken the lead and shown them other options. Now, whenever they go out to dinner with you, the expectation will be a light dessert or a warm cup of coffee and good conversation.

- This is only one example, and I know you will experience other ways to help those around you. **Remember that you can influence others by your actions and creative alternatives.**

CHAPTER 32
I BELIEVE IN YOU

"Change is not easy, but it is worth every moment. And I believe that you are worth every moment!"

Life comes with its ups and downs, and food is by your side throughout your journey. Recognize that food is meant to sustain you and is not a tool that controls you or comforts you. When you win the battle over food and establish a healthy, new relationship, food is no longer the adversary and becomes your partner.

STICKING TO YOUR GOALS
Because life is unpredictable, expect vulnerable moments when old thoughts may resurface. Don't revert to old habits like numbing yourself and aimlessly eating because these actions never create positive outcomes. The moment you feel stress, immediately stop to recognize what typically comes along with stress. Are the familiar feelings of guilt, disappointment, and selflessness rising to the surface again? If you answered, *"Yes,"* ask yourself, *"Do I want to feel that empty feeling as a result of my food choices?"* You know the answer is no because you want better for yourself. I know you can stick to your goals and keep food in your corner as an ally.

You are responsible for your actions and decisions. No one can fix or change you. Even though professionals can provide support and guidance and hold you accountable, you are ultimately responsible for your transformation. As your confidence increases, you will find that you can ride over bumps, make sharp turns, and act. I know you can continue to make forward progress with self-confidence and courage.

SEEING YOUR NEW REFLECTION

You've learned that how you think about food reflects how you see yourself. There may come times when you don't feel good about yourself and negative emotions rear their head. During these times, you may be tempted to grab a bag of chips and a soda – or worse. When this happens, take a breath and pause.

Don't let your inner voice justify food rewards. If you take enough "rewards," the result will be decreasing your health and wellbeing and gaining weight. And when are those rewards?

The moment you find yourself struggling, think about how your food choices reflect how you feel about yourself. Define how you feel at that moment and ask yourself, *"What are my options?" "Does dieting lead back to the negative mental thoughts and the weight cycle?" "Will procrastinating cause me to feel helpless again?"*

Remember that no one is perfect, and mistakes are part of being human. The key is to find solutions that prevent you from reverting to poor habits. I know that in time you will grow stronger, become more resilient, and be more comfortable as you continue to repeat the new processes.

What do you get in return? An entire shift in your perspective of how you see foods and more importantly, how you see yourself.

PARTING THOUGHTS

You are living your new truth. You know what held you back, and you know what you need to do in order to move forward. You are the priority! And you are the one who owns your success!

Go forward fearlessly. You will be successful because I believe in you, and because you now believe in yourself.